Reviews for Health and Weight Management –
Teachings From the East

"This is a refreshingly clear and easy to read explanation of eastern philosophy and health. It's full of practical applicable information and advice for optimum mental and physical wellness, (I loved it) everyone should have it as a reference point."

– *Marese McElduff, Lic Ac.*
Founder member of the Acupuncture Council of Ireland

"A timely and inspiring chronicle for the times we live in"

– *Frank Murphy, Tai Chi Instructor,*
7th Degree Black Belt, Master Instructor ITF, Taekwondo

"A clear, compassionate insightful read. This book is full of good information that gives down to earth explanations for a variety of Eastern practices as an aid to Western living."

Kevin Copeland

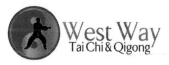

*This book is dedicated to my mother
Carmel Rainsford and to the memory of my late father
David Rainsford who were great teachers!*

Contents

Acknowledgements

....

I would like to acknowledge the support of my daughters Claire and Eleanor, my mother Carmel, Irene, David and Aidan and families and also my closest friends for all their encouragement.

I would also like to say special thanks to Marese McElduff Lic.Ac of The Regional Integrated Health Clinic and founding member of The Acupuncture Council of Ireland www.acupuncturecouncilofireland.com

I would also like to say special thanks to Kevin Copeland of Westway Tai chi and Qi Gong www.westway.ie, and to Frank Murphy of www.frankmurphysmasterclass.com.

Also to all at: www.taichiforhealthinstitute.org especially Dr Paul Lam and to all at www.taichicentre.com founded by Grandmaster Liming Yue.

Finally, I would like to say special thanks to Roger Sproston at www.straightforward.co.uk for all his support and encouragement to finish this book.

Disclaimer

The practices and remedies in this book are not a substitute for your doctor's advice. All matters in relation to your health require appropriate medical supervision. Neither the writer or publisher are engaged in giving professional advice to the reader.

While all efforts have been made to make sure that the information in this book is correct, it is possible that new research will supersede some of the information in this book. Neither the writer or the publisher will be liable for any alleged loss or damage from using the contents of this book.

While the writer has tried to ensure that the correct phone, web addresses and general addresses have been given, neither the writer nor the publisher will be responsible for any errors or changes that arise. Also the publisher has no control over or responsibility for the writer or third party websites.

Introduction

Health and Weight Management is all about stress and lifestyle management. Life circumstances such as stressful work, parenting, financial problems, divorce etc can throw us out of balance.

We can get completely caught up in one area of our lives to the detriment of the rest including our health and well-being. We may stop getting enough exercise, exist on a substandard diet and lose our sense of equilibrium. We need to take a virtual helicopter ride over our life to see what areas are red danger/stress zones and decide what we can do to make changes. Many people wait until they reach a health crisis before making changes but it is easier to start making changes now.

In the theory of Yin and Yang all things are constantly balancing and rebalancing. In the East there has been a tradition of mind body exercise since antiquity. The practice of Yoga in India dates back over 5,000 years. Tai Chi dates back 700 to 1500 years ago. Chinese Medicine in which the theory of Yin and Yang is central includes Acupuncture, Acupressure, Herbal medicine, Tai Chi and Qi Gong. One of the core beliefs is that the body's 'life force' or energy called Qi is circulating through channels called meridians in the body. These channels are linked to the organs of the body.

Western medicine is based on diagnosis. In Oriental Medicine, originating in China and practiced throughout the East in Japan, Korea and now worldwide, the treatment depends on the underlying imbalance. Illness and other emotional, mental and physical problems arise when the flow of Qi energy is weak or stagnated. Restoring the flow of Qi is crucial to balance yin and yang and to achieve health and wellness.

I include chapters on Self-Care, Emotions, Diet and Nutrition, Acupuncture and Acupressure, Tai Chi, Qi Gong, Herbs, Meditation, Lung health and Chinese Medicine theory. I have also written a chapter on Healthy Recipes and Remedies. Throughout the book I explain how Health and Weight Management go hand in hand. Health and Weight Management is not about punishing routines or diets, it is about finding a balance in our life, in physical activity, mind body exercise and food. In my chapter on Lung health, I examine how building Lung Qi is important in building resistance to infections and viruses.

In some of the major hospitals in China specialising in Western medicine, Traditional Chinese Medicine may also be offered. Many doctors in China who train in Western medicine take Traditional Chinese Medicine studies as part of their training. Western medicine and Traditional Chinese Medicine can be used at the same time and are complementary; helping to boost the immune system fight and prevent illness.

In Acupuncture and Medical Herbalism a clinical examination may include taking a family history of illness and the lifestyle of the client (especially work/life balance). More and more people are turning to Qi Gong, Acupuncture, Acupressure and Tai Chi to not only fight disease but to prevent it. Historically in the East, there is a more preventative approach to illness; a tradition of people going for treatment to keep well before becoming ill.

Tai chi and Qi Gong are mind body exercises which activate the flow of Qi in the body, removing blockages. By integrating acupuncture and acupressure in your wellness plan you will help maintain Qi energy flow.

The mind body connection has never been so relevant. In my chapter on Self-Care I deal with taking responsibility for self-care and developing awareness of our emotions.

On a personal note, my interest in the East started when I was a child. My uncle Joseph was a Chef with a passion for healthy food and travel. He lived in Australia and San Francisco for many years where he had Chinese friends from the food industry. He travelled in the East, writing to my mother from Japan. He also attended Yoga classes with Walt Baptiste, the famous yoga teacher in San Francisco. When he returned to Ireland he started a delicatessen business in Phibsboro, Dublin. I worked in his shop as a teenager and his interest in health and food made a huge impression on me.

My interest in Tai Chi started when I attended classes in my early 20's with Dr Deng (who was also an acupuncturist) off Grafton street in Dublin. I also got to know his wife who was learning English. They later returned to China. I have practiced both Yang and Chen styles of Tai Chi and Qi Gong and trained as an acupuncturist. I also trained as a Tai Chi instructor with Dr Paul Lam of the Tai Chi for Health Institute.

When you learn to cultivate self-awareness through the mind body exercises and meditation you will learn to value your mind and body and see your health as your wealth.

This is a lifetime's challenge, we can be doing well for a while but we can all slip back; we have to maintain a state of awareness to bring ourselves back into balance. Your health is your wealth!

"Love your neighbour as you love yourself"
— Mark 12:31

CHAPTER ONE

Self-Care

....

When our self-esteem is good we feel we can handle any-thing, we value and honour ourselves. We need to constantly choose our thoughts and our words. Positive thought patterns will attract positive energies. The best gift we can give ourselves in our lifetime is to recognise our own inherent value. When we develop an awareness of our own self-worth we will be able to live a more balanced and healthy lifestyle. Self-love and self-respect are essential for a healthy mind. The Latin phrase "mens sana in corpore sano" is translated as "a healthy mind in a healthy body."

We need to learn to programme our minds for health and wellness to help us achieve our life goals. If we turn to comfort food as a source of consolation, we need to instead find comfort and reassurance in self-care and by nourishing our bodies and our friendships.

Take a piece of paper and start by writing down all your positive points and all the good things you have going for you such as friends, your intelligence, a place to sleep etc. You will see that you have a lot more positives than you thought you had.

If we learn to see self-care as a priority, we will have more self-awareness as to how to prevent overload and burnout. You will begin to see sleep, a balanced diet and exercise as essential to health and well being. Self-awareness will build your confidence and lead to inner serenity and order.

Research has found that journaling for 15 to 20 minutes a day helps people to deal with traumatic, emotional and stressful situations.[1]

Self-care means developing good boundaries in your life; in asserting that your time for exercise/meal preparation is non- negotiable. In prioritising self-care you will learn to focus on what is really important and by doing what really matters to you. In deciding to prioritise self-care you will be choosing new exercise, relaxation and food planning habits.

You may be finding your work/ life balance is non-existent. The self-care and wellness practices rooted in Chinese Medicine centre on Qi or life force. We can practice self-care at home with acupressure and simple Qi Gong exercises. In Chinese Medicine, Yang Sheng means nourishing life. It is taking time to nourish your life inside and outside.

A Habit

> ... I am at your command
> Half the things you do well might just as well
> be turned over to me.
> For I can do them quickly, correctly and profitably
> I am easily managed, just be firm with me.
> Those who are great, I have made great.
> – Author unknown

Learning to punctuate your day with small meditation breaks will stop you getting stressed and off target. In Chinese medicine, Shen is translated as the "spirit" or "mind" and implies our consciousness, mental health, vitality and presence. We should try to nourish and develop an awareness of our Shen.

We need to adopt self-care rituals. Visualise yourself as your own best friend. Look in the mirror and tell yourself how much you appreciate and value yourself. A wise old grandmother used to tell her grandchildren "have a thought of yourself". Set your own boundaries and see yourself as valuable!

Creating the ritual of a home spa or visiting a spa or swimming pool is a part of Japanese culture that we could emulate. In Japan, water is regarded as the symbol of life, always flowing, changing and renewing. Immersion in water allows the body to rest, restore and revive.

We have to move away from neglecting our care needs. A self-care mindset is maintaining a frame of mind that "It is essential to take care of myself."

We could look at the maintenance of the human body as similar to maintaining a car. If we supply the engine with good quality fuel or energy, we must also supply our bodies with the best quality nutrition and Food Qi. In Chinese medicine the spleen sends Food Qi (energy) to our lungs; careful choice of nutrition and good digestion will help respiration.

Our goals for self-care should be improved physical fitness, a reduction in stress, improved nutrition and a balance between work and personal life. Self-care is important in developing resilience. Self-compassion helps us to take care of ourselves better. By recognising our own worth and value we can achieve balance and happiness. Self-acceptance and self- love are essential to our mental health.

Having a "running away day" every one/ two months will pay you dividends. Every one to two months I will drive to the coast and walk, rejuvenating the mind. The world won't stop if you aren't around for a few hours. We must see health and well-being as a form of preventative medicine. In China and in the East, patients will go for acupuncture before an illness gets established. The classic Chinese text – *The Nei Jing*, explains the wisdom of preventative medicine.[2]

"The sages of antiquity did not treat those who were already sick but those who were not sick...". – *Nei Jing*

The degree of success we have in any endeavour, in improving our health or weight management will be guided by our self-image. When we have a good self-image we attract more positive results. The relationship you have with yourself is the most important one you will ever have.

The way to open the door to success is to visualise it and see ourselves as being successful. Self-hypnosis helps you make suggestions to the subconscious mind for lasting results.

You can change negative thoughts to positive ones by constant repetition, keep believing and persevering. By constantly reaffirming your positive self-image, your subconscious will learn to establish positive core beliefs. You must see yourself as moving towards your goal with confidence.

Faith
Faith has been shown to improve well being. The National Opinion Research Centre (NORC) in the USA in 1984 collected research on church attendance and happiness. The data demonstrated a positive relationship between faith and happiness.[3] The book "The Power of Positive Thinking"

by Norman Vincent Peale first published in 1952 is still an international bestseller.[4]

> "Believe in yourself! Have faith in your abilities! Without a humble but reasonable confidence in your own powers you cannot be successful or happy."
> – Norman Vincent Peale

> "Many of life's failures are people who did not realise how close they were to success when they gave up."
> – Thomas Edison

> "It is your opinion of and value of yourself that matters, not anyone else's!"　　　　　　　　　– Anonymous

Intuition

We all need to tap into our intuition and inner wisdom. Intuition is not logical. We need to develop awareness to help us listen to our intuitive voice. Listen to your inner guide. When you meditate, take a deep breath and relax and you will find it easier to tap into your intuition. The Chinese writing character for crisis is also the character for opportunity. We can see our difficulties as an opportunity for change and growth.

Benefits of Self-Care

Self-Care – prevents the negative effects of stress

Self-Care – prevents us from burning out

Self-Care – helps us to plan

Self-Care – helps us to reset and refocus

Self-Care – is taking care of our emotional and physical needs

Self-Care – is healthy nutrition and exercise

Self-Care – is taking structured times every day for mind-body exercise, to meditate, practice Tai Chi, Qi Gong or Yoga.

Self-Kindness

Self-kindness is being gentle with ourselves when there are setbacks. We can wipe the slate clean and start again at any time of the day. Planning structured times for food shopping, food preparation, exercise and mind- body practice will make it easier to keep ourselves on the right track.

Taking time to plan will make us more productive in the long run. Being our own best friend helps us to accept and nourish the whole that is us. There are times we have to clear away emotional baggage to make space for new and healthier choices. We can address these issues with a therapist. What would you say to a good friend who was going through a hard time? You would say "give yourself a break", say the same to yourself!

Ways to Build Your Power
1. Decide you are in the Driving seat of your life
2. Have faith in your own power and wisdom
3. Plan your goals to make changes
4. Believe in your intuition
5. Go get it !

> "Every living cell in your body is eavesdropping on your mind"   – Deepak Chopra

> "Slow down and get there more productively"
>   – Author Unknown

Intentions and Affirmations
I nurture my mind, spirit and body daily.
I honour my body with self-care, healthy food, meditation and exercise.
I celebrate myself.
I am renewed and re-energised.

Getting in Touch with your Desires

What are my core values?

What do I need to do to get my life in balance with my values?

Do I give myself permission to get what I want?

Simplify your life, take a look at how much energy you spend chasing things you don't need.

Self-Care in Japan.

In Japan there is a concept called Mie-nai Oshareh which means unseen beauty. It is believed that true beauty comes from inside. A study examined the prevalence of self-care, sources of self-care information and reasons for self-care in the UK, USA, Australia and Japan, the result showed the prevalence of self-care was highest in Japan at 54%.[5]

"A smile will gain you ten more years of life"
– Chinese Proverb

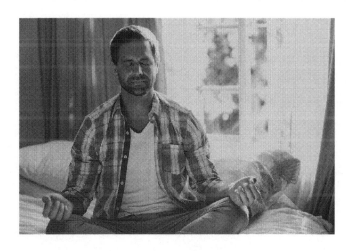

11

CHAPTER TWO

Emotions

In the west we do not generally realise how our emotions affect our general health and well-being. An emotion is defined as a strong feeling deriving from one's circumstances, mood or relationships with others.

In Traditional Chinese medicine, our emotions are linked to the meridians which are the pathways through which our Qi energy flows. Different emotions are linked to the heart, lungs, spleen, liver and kidneys.

The emotion associated with the heart is joy. The emotion associated with the lungs is grief, excess worry is linked to the spleen, anger is linked to the liver and the kidneys are associated with fear. When our emotions flow easily in response to different situations our Qi energy flows smoothly and we maintain good health. However, when a single emotion dominates, our internal energies stagnate and we become prone to ill health.[1]

> "It is known that all diseases arise from the upset of Qi. Anger pushes the Qi up, joy makes the Qi slacken, grief disperses the Qi, fear brings the Qi down, terror confuses the Qi and anxiety causes the Qi to stagnate."
>
> – *The Nei Jing*

Table of Emotions[2]

Anger (including repressed anger and irritability)	Joy (including over-excitement) Over-excitement over a long time can affect the heart	Grief (including sadness and excessive melancholy)	Worry (including excessive thinking and excessive mental work can affect spleen energy)	Fear (including deep shock)
Anger affects the liver resulting in stagnation of liver Qi	Over-excitement is connected to symptoms of insomnia, palpitations and unease	Excessive grief and melancholy weaken the lungs	Eating irregularly or mindlessly and too quickly will throw the digestion out of balance	In cases of extreme fear and fright, the kidneys ability to hold Qi is affected
Anger can affect the stomach, the spleen and the liver	Joy makes the mind peaceful and relaxed, The heart is associated with joy	Sadness depletes Qi. The lungs govern Qi	Excessive worry weakens spleen energy	Too much fear and fright weakens kidney energy

Emotions can affect our health and judgment, Aristotle 384–322 BC described emotions "as all those feelings that so change men as to affect their judgement". We would not be fully alive without them, but there are times in our lives when one or more emotions can become out of balance. We need to develop an awareness of our thoughts by weeding out negative thought patterns.

If we are going through emotional pain whether from the past or the present, we should acknowledge and process the pain through counselling or journaling.

If we don't, the buried emotion will keep on eating at us. Whenever we avoid something it will usually manifest in more problems and could lead to using food or other addictions in an effort to deny the problem. It is wiser and healthier to deal with the feelings of loss or grief, fear, guilt or loneliness etc. at source rather than allow them to develop into a more serious health problem.

A number of years ago a client came to see me who was substantially overweight, she also suffered with associated health problems. When we started taking a case history, she told me she had tried a variety of slimming clubs and therapists and she was not happy with her experience. When I told her it would take a number of therapy sessions and changes to her current food and exercise routine she became agitated. She was seeking a quick fix solution.

While there is no quick fix solution you can make an improvement every day. Emile Coué, the French psychologist who developed the Coué method of autosuggestion recommended repeating to yourself "Every day in every way, I'm getting better and better" preferably as many as twenty times a day, especially every morning and evening.[3]

Food Addictions

For some people food can become an addiction. Food like drink, drugs and gambling can become a way to mask difficult feelings. An article in *Scientific American* in March 2010 by Katherine Harmon noted that a study in which rats were given access to high fat foods showed some of the same characteristics as animals hooked on cocaine or heroin.[4]

Social Media

Our minds and bodies are becoming increasingly disconnected with over-reliance on social media. We could learn from the East where the importance of union in mind and body is recognised. The practice of Tai Chi, Yoga, Qi Gong and meditation develop the mind body connection. In Chinese medicine when our Shen ("spirit" or "mind") is healthy, we have good vitality.

> "The secret of health for both mind and body is not to mourn for the past, nor to worry about the future, but to live the present moment wisely and earnestly."
>
> – The Buddha

The Limbic System

The Limbic System is a set of structures of the brain. They are located on both sides of the Thalamus beneath the cerebrum. The limbic system governs our sleep cycles, appetite, libido etc. If the limbic system gets thrown out of balance through excess stress, it can make self-control of our mood and appetite more difficult. By understanding the link between stress and overeating, we can learn to take preventative measures by strengthening the mind body connection and Qi.

Chinese medicine teaches us that balance is the key to good health, i.e. balance in diet, in rest, exercise and in our emotional life.[5]

Affirmations

By programming your mind for health through visualisation you will actualise your health goals.

A client who was trying to lose weight and get fit was stuck in a negative mindset. With positive self-affirmations she stopped criticising herself and began replacing her negative self-talk with positive affirmations such as "today will be a better day" and "I will eat healthily today." Over time she lost the weight she wanted to lose and her overall health improved. We must recognise our self-worth. If we do not love ourselves, we keep the best away from us.

Research has now linked the direct neurological connections between the brain and the immune system. Many hospitals and treatment centres recommend relaxation, meditation and visualisation classes. Psychoneuroimmunology is the study of the interactions between human behaviour, the neural, endocrine and immune processes.

The 1991 book *Psychoneuroimmunology*, edited by Ader, Cohen and Felton reports studies on the relationship between the nervous and immune systems.[6]

Hormones and Stress

Our hormonal system reacts to stress with the release of hormones. The stress hormones slow the body's metabolism and encourage the storage of fat.

The two main stress hormones are cortisol and adrenaline which are produced by the adrenals and are two small glands situated above the kidneys. Adrenaline affects the autonomous nervous system that controls the heart rate, dilation of pupils, perspiration and saliva.

In stressful situations the adrenaline that is released enables you to stay alert and focused while the hormone cortisol increases the levels of fat and sugar in the bloodstream. After a period of stress adrenaline levels return to normal in a short time but cortisol levels remain elevated.

A study of older adults has shown that Qi Gong reduces cortisol secretion.[7] If you do not exercise during a period of stress, all the extra energy from the fat and sugar has no purpose and will become fat. Excess stress hormones encourage the storage of the hardest-to-shift weight, which is around the abdomen.

We are aware that excess body fat contributes to heart attacks, strokes, high blood pressure, cancer and diabetes;

but scientists have recognised that excess abdominal fat is dangerous. Abdominal fat cells have more receptors for cortisol.[8]

A study presented to the European Society for Cardiology said that the location of fat is just as important as the amount of it. Adults with normal mass index (BMI) and extra belly fat (termed "central obesity") had a 79% higher risk of major cardiovascular events compared with people who were mildly overweight but with normal fat distribution.[9]

If the stress levels continue, the cortisol levels remain elevated and blood sugar increases. If the body is stressed out too often, you can become insulin resistant. Insulin resistance can cause an increased risk of diabetes and heart disease.

Single parents, both men and women may be prone to high levels of stress in trying to combine work, family, finances and housework. Because of this, they may have to take extra care to manage stress by taking time for themselves to practice meditation and other mind body exercises.

For women who are planning on becoming pregnant; it may be safer to lose some excess weight beforehand. Some women are insulin resistant during pregnancy and a small percentage end up with temporary gestational diabetes.

For women in perimenopause and menopause, the body is slower to let go of fat around the middle as fat cells make oestrogen. Testosterone levels drop with age and muscle mass shrinks, so without a conscious effort to stay fit it will be harder to burn off fat. High stress levels resulting in high cortisol levels cause reduced levels of T3 the thyroid hormone, this is not good as T3 is the thyroid hormone that burns fat.[10]

High levels of stress weakens the immune systems gut barrier and can lead to "leaky gut" releasing undigested food particles and bacteria into the bloodstream which can cause chronic inflammation. The gut barrier provides a strong defence and plays a pivotal role in the link between the gut microbiota and the immune system.[11]

By reducing our stress and cortisol levels, we will also reduce oxidation in the body and premature ageing of the cells. Chronic inflammation breaks down collagen which is the protein that keeps skin firm, plump and smooth resulting in fine lines and dryness.

> "Unmet needs create stress and stress produces toxic hormones, such as cortisol."
> – Christine Northrup, M.D.

Chronic stress over a prolonged period causes blockages and imbalances in the body. We may not even be aware that our default system is constant worry. We need to break the pattern by changing old habits through meditation and mind body exercise like Qi Gong, Tai Chi and yoga.

Microbiota

Stress damages the level of good bacteria in the gut. An example is Candida Albicans; when this is out of control, it causes food cravings, fatigue, bloated stomach and brain fog. Our gut also acts as a barrier to invading organisms. Up to 70% of the immune system is in our gut.[12]

UCLA has done work on how trillions of bacteria in the gut communicate with the enteric nervous system cells. Dr Purna Kashyap, a gastroenterologist at the Mayo Clinic in Rochester, Minnesota says that gut bacteria are likely to be an important determinant of the degree of weight loss attained following lifestyle and dietary intervention.[13]

A study of 292 people found that those who were over-weight had lower gut bacteria diversity and higher levels of c-reactive protein, an inflammatory marker in the blood.[14] Research has also found that exposure to a social stressor alters the structure of the intestinal microbiota.[15]

Japan has one of the lowest obesity levels in the world and is known for the long life spans of its people especially in Okinawa. The secret could lie in the Japanese diet. Japanese and Korean diets are balanced and have fermented and probiotic rich foods which are good for gut microbiota.

Self-Referral

Dr Deepak Chopra in his book, Perfect Digestion discusses a process that is known in Ayurveda as self-referral. This means looking within to help in decision making. He says "We must begin by placing our attention on our internal cues." He also says we need to develop an awareness that every emotion includes both a thought and a physical feeling and when upset we should close our eyes and our mind will be attracted to an area in the body. We should then allow our attention to rest on that area for a short while and gradually the physical sensation will moderate; on opening our eyes the emotional element will also have diminished.[16]

Self-awareness helps us to make wise decisions such as reducing overwork; meditation improves awareness.

Sleep

When we are tired, we are more prone to being out of balance emotionally. We could all benefit with structured times for relaxation and rest to maintain physical and emotional balance. Our "grandparents adage that every hour of sleep before midnight is worth two after midnight may have some truth" according to Dr Matt Walker, head of the sleep and neuroimaging lab at the university of California, Berkeley. He says "our sleep quality changes as the night wears on, that non-REM sleep dominates slumber cycles in the early part of the night, but as the clock moves towards daybreak, REM sleep becomes predominant". Research has suggested that non-REM sleep is deeper and more restorative than lighter dream infused REM sleep but he says "both types offer benefits".[17]

Sleep deprivation can result in weight gain. Sleep and the lack of sleep affect the nightly hormones which are ghrelin and leptin. Ghrelin is the hormone that tells you when to eat; when sleep deprived, we have more ghrelin. Leptin tells us to stop eating, when we are sleep deprived we have less leptin. Regular structured times for sleep help to restore our energy and maintain emotional equilibrium.

How To Improve Sleep
1. Reduce tea, cola and caffeine before bedtime.
2. By eating every three to four hours our adrenaline levels will remain steady and the hormone cortisol will start to wind down if we go to bed at a reasonable time.
3. Try to get some exercise a few hours before bed time to unwind.
4. Practice some meditation, Tai Chi, Qi Gong or Yoga in the evening time.

Spirit
By strengthening our connection to the higher power of God, helps improve peace, calmness and reassurance.

Take Time to Eat

When you are hungry for emotional comfort, food won't quench the emotional appetite. Switch activity straight away and go for a walk, put on some music and dance or phone a friend. For improved digestion do not drink much fluid at meal time and drink more fluid between meals. Excess fluids with meals can dilute the digestive juices making them less effective.

Tips for Stress and Emotional Eating

1. Make a weekly meal plan.
2. Do a twice weekly shop.
3. Exercise everyday.
4. Prioritise your time.
5. Build in relaxation periods in your day to meditate, read, do some gardening or chill!

Exercise

> "Exercise would cure a guilty conscience."
>
> – Plato

Studies show that exercise can reduce the impact of stress. The mental benefits of aerobic exercise also have a neurochemical basis. Exercise reduces the levels of adrenaline and cortisol and it stimulates the production of endorphins, which are natural analgesics and mood elevators.[18]

> "If you do not change direction, you may end up where you are heading".
>
> – Lao Tzu

CHAPTER THREE

Diet and Nutrition

....

"Let food be your medicine and medicine be your food."
– Hippocrates

In Chinese medicine our diet and nutrition are integral in the whole body approach to health.

"When the body is imbalanced, the physician should use dietetics to harmonise and fortify. The five grains are used to nourish, the five fruits to assist, the five animals to fortify, the five vegetables to fulfil. Combining the energetic properties of these in one's diet can reinforce the essence and energy."
– *The Yellow Emperor's Classic of Medicine*

We eat food to promote the energy flow (Qi) of the body and to improve health and vitality. So it is important to obtain good nutrition. The middle Jiao or abdomen in the body is the area where digestion takes place.

Dampness and Stagnation

In traditional Chinese medicine, it is believed that certain foods make our internal systems damp, phlegmy or sluggish. These symptoms start off in the liver, digestive system and spleen causing stagnation to the rest of the body. Stagnation causes weight gain, bloating, low energy and phlegmy lungs. The spleen sends Food-Qi up to the lungs. Too much dampness can contribute to yeast infections and joint inflammation.

Food should be cooked lightly to retain minerals and vitamins. Steaming vegetables is the best way to retain nutrients. Overcooking food in too much fat and oil can lead to the accumulation of internal damp and phlegm which damages the spleens ability to assist digestion. Spleen energy is improved with some warming foods and by not over consuming cold raw foods. Over-consumption of hot spicy foods can damage the energy flow (Qi).[1]

Our selection of food should take cognisance of the energetic qualities of foods such as cooling, drying, warming or lubricating. We should seek to cool the heat, warm the cold, dry the dampness and lubricate the dryness.

Dietary Tips:
1. Too much dairy products especially cheese and milk produce dampness and should be avoided.
2. Steam or lightly cook vegetables to maintain nutrients.
3. Avoid cooking in heavy fats or oils.
4. Sweet food, soda drinks and coffee should be kept to a minimum.
5. Consume raw foods in moderation.
6. Fatty, greasy foods cause stagnation.
7. Chew food slowly, at least 22 times for each bite.

Chewing and Savouring
Research published in the *American Journal of Clinical Nutrition* said eating more slowly could be a simple way of tackling weight management. Results from the research showed that

overweight participants chewed less and ate more quickly than lean ones. The research was carried out at the Harbin Medical University in China.[2]

Chewing is a major part of digestion. The digestive process begins in the mouth where enzymes are produced to help break down and absorb nutrients. When chewing, slow down, savour the flavour and texture of your food, enjoy!

Before you start eating, take a couple of seconds to settle your mind and breathe deeply. If you eat while emotionally upset, you are more likely to cause indigestion and hinder the energy flow (Qi). Try to eat at the kitchen table, if at home; as it can help you to be more mindful of what you are eating.

Five Smaller Meals
Five smaller meals a day will keep the blood sugar more stable. Eating approximately every three hours will help keep appetite under control, boost the metabolism and reduce cortisol. When you switch to eating little and often you will notice that you can maintain your energy levels; as your blood sugar level is stable, your energy levels will also be stable and there will be less roller-coaster highs and lows. Also when the blood sugar level is steady, your body will be less likely to look for a quick fix of sugar.

Breakfast: Could include porridge or home-made muesli and a fruit or vegetable smoothie.

Mid-Morning: Fruit/seeds or a smoothie.

Lunch: Steamed vegetables, potatoes or brown rice and fish, meat or chicken. Alternatively a salad, a warm salad is preferable in cold weather. Another option is a home-made chicken/turkey/meat sandwich with salad and home-made soup which can also be brought to work in a flask/food warmer.

Mid Afternoon: Nuts, seeds or fruit. A trail mix of almonds, nuts, pumpkin, sesame and sunflower seeds helps to keep the blood sugar even.

Dinner: Small stir fry with lots of vegetables (and little oil) or steamed vegetables and potatoes/brown rice and fish. Alternatively, home-made soup which is a fantastic option as it can also serve as lunch the next day.

Try to not eat after 7pm as it can cause acid reflux and to always eat breakfast. It is better if meals decrease in size throughout the day to ensure that all food is well digested before sleeping. By substituting tea for coffee you are lowering cortisol levels and increasing antioxidants.

In Japan, Hara Hachi Bu means eating until you are 80% full. The Okinawan people in Japan (many of whom live to be centenarians) are known to practice Hara Hachi Bu. There is a Japanese proverb that says "Eight parts of a full stomach sustain the man; the other two sustain the doctor."

The *Nei Jing* (an ancient Chinese medical text) says "If no food eaten for half a day Qi is weakened, if no food is eaten for a day Qi is depleted." This shows that early Chinese medicine did not favour fasting.

Temperature and Flavour
Food is classified by temperature and flavour in Traditional Chinese Medicine. When we are healthy and strong we can better tolerate a variety of food. If we are weak and unwell we should eat more warming foods like soups and stews.

If you overheat easily and have a dry mouth, cooling foods like cucumber, watermelon, peppermint and cold salads may be better for you.

If you are inclined to be cold and tire easily, warming foods like ginger, chicken and pumpkin are good. Cooler foods like raw fruit and vegetables are good during hotter weather. Animal foods such as poultry and meat are warming and fruit, raw vegetables and liquids cool us. Beans, deep sea fish, legumes, seeds and nuts are neutral. The hot and excessive type of person would be better limiting animal products while the cold and deficient type would benefit from having more warming foods.[3]

Over-consumption of sugar is to be avoided. Not only does sugar increase weight gain but it can also cause inflammation, degeneration and disease. In Chinese medicine eating too many sweet foods may cause problems of internal heat and impairment of spleen function, it can also affect kidney Qi. When we overeat, we stress our digestive system and produce more toxins and waste products.[4]

"From the viewpoint of Chinese medicine, moderation, discipline and balance are the fundamental concepts to bear in mind when considering eating. Be aware of the flavours and temperature of the food, be aware of a disciplined approach to quiet and reflective eating and be aware of the body's natural daily rhythms."
– Tom Williams PhD

Acid – Alkaline Balance
Our acid alkaline balance is very important for good digestion. The pH is the measurement of the acid to alkaline ratio. It ranges from 1.0 – very acidic to 14.0 – very alkaline. Our blood pH should be a little alkaline at about 7.3 to 7.4.

Readings above and below this can lead to ill health. The body is constantly trying to balance its pH. Research has shown that a long term acidic diet can result in inflammation and can also cause premature ageing and free radical damage.

A diet that is heavy in animal fat, caffeine and sugar strains the body's ability to maintain pH neutrality. It can also run down the body's store of alkaline minerals such as magnesium, potassium and calcium, which are essential for good health.

It is good to select plenty of alkaline foods such as vegetables, fruits, nuts, seeds and grains such as millet and quinoa and to eat less acidic food such as meat, sugar, caffeine and dairy. Our diet should be a balance of complex carbohydrates, protein, whole grains and fish, vegetables, fruit, nuts and seeds. Try and replace white rice and pasta with brown rice, millet and buckwheat. Foods such as broccoli, kale, spinach and asparagus are chlorophyll rich.[5]

Tips:
Drinking warm water with squeezed lemon helps reduce fluid retention and drains dampness in the body. Taking digestive enzymes can improve our digestion if suffering from indigestion or acid reflux.

Eliminating and Cutting Down Sugars and Refined Carbohydrates
Sugar can lead to insulin resistance and causes weight gain around the abdomen. Sugar can be found in tinned vegetables, tomato ketchup, baked beans, yogurts and tinned soups. Slow releasing carbohydrates are more beneficial.[6]

Slow Releasing Carbohydrates	Fast Releasing Carbohydrates
Rye, oats, brown rice, millet and quinoa	White bread, white flour, pastries, biscuits
Lentils and beans	Sugar and honey
Vegetables	Potatoes
Fruit	Dried fruit, fruit juice and grapes

Wheat

Wheat contains gluten which is a protein. The gluten forms a sticky substance in the digestive system. Because it is difficult to digest, it can produce gas.

Too Few Carbohydrates

Just as fast releasing carbohydrates cause problems, too few carbohydrates can also cause problems; the blood sugar plummets and the body releases adrenaline to help raise blood glucose and may cause high cortisol levels.

Adding Protein to Every Meal

As the muscles are made up of protein, we need to make sure that we are getting enough protein to keep muscle mass. We should add protein to each meal. When we add protein to a carbohydrate, it changes to a slow releasing carbohydrate. You can do this for example by adding nuts and seeds to porridge.

When we keep eating foods that our body finds difficult to digest, we continue to boost our cortisol levels and increase our tendency to store fat. Examples of this are wheat, dairy, chocolate, sugar and caffeine.[7]

Seaweed and Fish

Seaweed contains iodine which is important for the thyroid gland which regulates our metabolism. Various types of seaweed include Nori, Kombu and Agar. Carrigeen moss is a seaweed which is found off the south and west coasts of Ireland. It is used to treat coughs and colds. It is rich in iodine and trace elements and is full of natural gelatine. The word Carigeen is "little rock" in Gaelic.

Essential fatty acids are nutrients that the body can't produce itself. We can only get these nutrients through diet or supplements. Essential fatty acids help to lose abdominal fat by reversing insulin resistance. EFA's also reduce inflammation. The body uses an enzyme to convert Omega 6 EFA's to GLA and Omega 3 to EPA and DHA; however this process gets interrupted by stress hormones and insulin, so it is very important to work at stress reduction. Omega 3 is found in flaxseeds, walnuts, green leafy vegetables, oily fish and pumpkin seeds. Omega 6 is found in sunflower seeds, sesame seeds, almonds and cashews.[8]

Drinks

Water is important for the whole body. It is essential for circulation, excretion and absorption. We should aim to drink 6–8 glasses of water a day. The human body is made up of more than 70% water. Herbal teas help to increase your liquid intake.

Drinks to avoid: all shop bought fruit juices, coffee, colas, sodas and drinks with artificial sweeteners. Caffeine may lower your insulin sensitivity. Alcohol consumption over an extended period causes cortisol to be released and can gradually cause insulin resistance.

Japanese Diet

The traditional Japanese diet uses more fish, portions of rice and lots of vegetables, pickled and fermented food. It generally has a lower overall sugar intake. The Traditional Japanese and Korean diet has fermented and probiotic rich food, which improve gut microbiota.

The protective action of lactic acid producing foods was pointed out in a study of Japanese Americans, by J.S. Clarke and was published in the Western Journal of Medicine. Clarke found that Americans of Japanese descent still living on their traditional Japanese diet, including about two tablespoons of miso per day and their traditional fermented foods, had a significantly different population of microbes compared with average Americans.[9]

In Japan an ichiju-sansai meal is a balanced meal. This is a combination of soup and three other dishes with rice and pickled vegetables always included. A main dish will generally comprise of protein rich foods like fish, egg or tofu and grains, vegetables, beans, mushrooms, seaweed etc providing minerals, fibre and vitamins. The soup is usually a variation of miso soup and the three side dishes are generally one protein based dish and two vegetable based dishes. Many Japanese households will have a rice cooker.

The Japanese diet encourages mindful eating. You can't easily eat an ichiju-sansai style meal on the couch. The variety of dishes and food types are central to eating in a manner that supports healthy habits. There is scientific reasoning behind mindful eating. The parasympathetic state helps to digest food properly. We need the nervous system to be in "rest and digest mode" for the salivary glands to release the enzyme amylase which is needed to begin the chemical breakdown of starches. The parasympathetic state also signals the pancreas

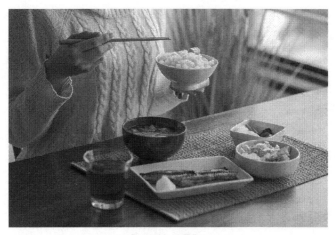

Japanese Diet

into secreting digestive enzymes to complete the breakdown of food in the small intestine. When we are under stress our bodies can't break down the food we have eaten and absorb the nutrients and we may get signals that we are still hungry and start overeating.

The lesson of ichiju-sansei is that we can enjoy food by paying attention to how and what we eat.

Sushi: A Japanese dish of vinegared rice together with a variety of ingredients such as seafood and vegetables.

Miso: Miso is fermented soybean. It has beneficial bacteria and antioxidants and is a complete protein containing all the essential amino acids. It is commonly eaten in soup.

Miso Soup: A traditional Japanese soup consisting of Dashi(stock) into which miso paste is mixed. A variety of ingredients can be added.

Tamari: A Japanese version of soy sauce. The main difference being that it contains little or no wheat (check the label).

Tamari is usually darker and has a less salty taste then soy sauce.

Nori: This is a type of edible seaweed from the red algae Genus Pryopia. It is generally used in Japanese cuisine for wrapping rolls of sushi

Kombu: Kombu is kelp and is widely eaten in east Asia. Okinawan cuisine uses a lot of Kombu in cooking, it is iodine rich.

Wakame: It is a species of edible seaweed and has a distinct flavour and texture. It is most often used in soups and salads.

Green Tea and Chi
Green Tea: It is made from Camellia Sinensis leaves and buds without the same withering and oxidation process that is used to make oolong teas and black tea. Green tea originated in China but has spread to many other Asian countries and worldwide. It is loaded with polyphenol antioxidants and contains the amino acid L-theanine which boosts the metabolic rate and can increase fat burning. Green tea contains catechins which may prevent the growth of bacteria and certain viruses. Green tea may cause mild reductions in blood sugar levels and helps with weight loss.

Sencha Tea: A type of Japanese Ryokucha and is made by infusing the processed whole tea leaves in hot water and is the commonest type of Japanese green tea.

Matcha Tea: It is rich in catechins, these are plant compounds which are natural antioxidants. By adding matcha powder to hot water, the tea will contain the nutrients from the entire leaf. It is also said to help with memory.

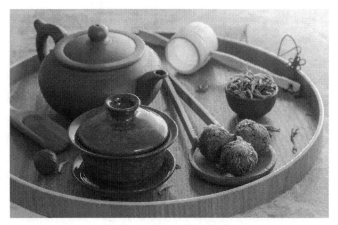

Green Tea and Chi

Jasmine Tea: It is scented with Jasmine blossoms. It will generally have green tea as the tea base.

Bancha Tea: It is from the same tree as Sencha but is gathered later and gets a lower market grade.

Summary for Healthy Eating
1. Do not eat when stressed or distracted. Chew your food slowly.
2. Eat sitting down and mindfully. Try to not eat after 7pm.
3. Snack on trail mix of raisins, seeds, and nuts. Carry this around with you so there is less temptation to reach for sugary foods. You can also use low fat hummus as a dip for vegetable snacks.
4. Drink warm water and lemon to reduce fluid retention.
5. Substitute herbal, green and black teas for coffee.
6. Avoid sweet foods and soda drinks as much as possible.
7. Eat five smaller meals a day.
8. Aim for a balanced diet of protein, complex carbohydrates, wholegrain, nuts, vegetables and fruit.

9. Try to increase chlorophyll rich food such a kale, broccoli, spinach, dandelion greens and asparagus. By eating plenty of fresh fruit and vegetables we are supplying our body with age-reversing antioxidants.
10. Avoid greasy, fried, spicy and heavy starchy foods which cause stagnation.
11. Limit dairy foods as they produce dampness and mucus.
12. A major cause of excessive weight gain is lack of exercise. A healthy diet and exercise is the key to a healthy metabolism.
13. Instead of looking to food for comfort, seek nourishment from building good relationships and by being thankful.
14. See food as fuel. You would only use the best quality fuel/energy for your car, do likewise for your body.
15. Include protein with every meal.
16. Use brown rice, millet, oats and quinoa instead of white rice and pasta.

An important part of Japanese food culture is to thank everything and everyone involved in the preparation of the meal including the waiter, the chef and the food itself. The phrase itadakimasu is used before a meal. This expression of gratitude comes from the verb itadaku which means to receive.

CHAPTER FOUR

Chinese Medicine

....

"Yin and Yang are the laws of heaven and earth, the great
framework of everything, the parents of change, the root
and beginning of life and death..."
                                  – The Book of Plain Questions

In Chinese medicine Yin and Yang are separate entities with
opposing natures.

Different parts of the body are either Yin or Yang. The
Qi of the body that is responsible for moving and warming
functions is Yang while the Qi of the body that is responsible
for nourishing and moistening functions is Yin.[1]

The different natures of Yin and Yang result in a power
struggle to dominate each other e.g. heat which is Yang
might dispel cold while cold which is Yin might lower the
temperature. In normal circumstances and conditions in the
body a balance is maintained through the opposing natures
of Yin and Yang.[2]

Yin and Yang
In this picture the white colour is Yang
and the black colour is Yin. The opposite
natures of Yin and Yang are shown by
the curved line which illustrates the inter-
consuming and supporting relationship.

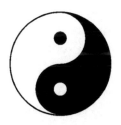

The white Yang space has a black spot (Yin) and the black Yin area has a white spot (Yang) showing the potential for change and transformation.[3]

Harmony and Balance
The root cause of the occurrence of ill health is the imbalance of Yin and Yang. The basic principle and purpose of acupuncture, acupressure, Tai Chi and Qi Gong is to adjust Yin and Yang and to re-establish harmony and balance in the body. The pull that takes place between Yin and Yang creates the energy which nourishes nature and human life.[4] Traditional Chinese medicine categorises every part of the body as either mainly Yin or Yang and good health is achieving a balance between the two.[5]

Case History
A woman of 50 was complaining of coldness, tiredness and weight gain. She had a weak pulse and pale and swollen tongue. She was presenting with spleen yang deficiency with internal dampness resulting in increased weight. Acupuncture was used to treat the spleen Yang deficiency.

Excesses and Deficiencies
We are all a combination of Yin and Yang. All parts of the body are either mainly Yin or Yang. Where there is an excess of Yin there will be a deficiency of Yang and the symptoms may include slow pulse, tiredness and coldness. We may prefer gentler exercise. When there is an excess of Yang there will be a deficiency of Yin, symptoms could include excessive sweating and thirst. We might be more inclined towards strenuous workouts.[6]

What causes the excesses and deficiencies? It is the

movement of Qi which is a fundamental concept of Chinese medicine.

The Functions of Qi

The functions of Qi are transforming, holding, transporting, raising, protecting and warming. Qi has been translated as "energy" or "life-force".[7] The development of the human body, the zang fu organs, the meridians and the circulation of blood are all dependent on Qi.[8]

Qi takes various forms in the body and fulfils a variety of functions.

The Types of Qi

1. Original Qi. (Yuan Qi) This is essence in the form of Qi. It originates in the kidneys.

2. Food Qi. (Gu Qi). Food when it enters the stomach is transformed into Food Qi by the spleen. Food Qi is extracted from food and is the starting point for creation of Qi and blood, it explains why Chinese medicine gives such importance to the quality of the food that we eat.

3. Gathering Qi (Zong Qi) Gathering Qi results from the interaction of Food Qi with air. The spleen sends Food Qi up to the lungs where along with air, it is transformed into Gathering Qi.

4. True Qi (Zhen Qi) This is the last stage of the transformation of Qi. It is the Qi which circulates in the meridians and nourishes our organs.

5. Nutritive Qi or Ying Qi. This is nutritive or nourishing Qi. Nutritive Qi nourishes the whole body and the organs. Nutritive Qi is extracted from food and water.

6. Defensive Qi or Wei Qi. Wei means to protect. In chapter 43 of the Chinese book, "Simple Questions"; it says

"Defensive Qi is derived from the course part of food and water". It protects the body from exterior factors such as wind, cold, heat and damp. It warms and nourishes the skin and muscles.[9]

Disharmonies of Qi
1. Deficient Qi – This is where there is insufficient Qi to carry out the different functions.
2. Sinking Qi – If the Qi is deficient it may no longer perform the holding function and sinks.
3. Stagnant Qi – When normal Qi is affected there may be blockages of Qi and sluggish movement.
4. Rebellious Qi – This is when Qi is flowing in the wrong direction.[10]

Jing
Jing in Chinese medicine is usually translated as essence. The word essence is used in three different categories: 1) Pre-heaven essence 2) Post-heaven essence and 3) Kidney essence.

Pre-heaven essence is inherited from our parents. The best way to conserve our Pre-heaven essence is to have a balance between work and rest, good diet and exercise. Post-heaven essence originates from food. Kidney essence originates in the kidneys but circulates all over the body.

When the essence and Qi are healthy, the mind will be happy and balanced and we will be more likely to have good health.[11]

Shen
Chinese medicine sees the heart as the home of the mind (Shen).[12] This is the mind or spirit of the individual. If the heart energy is strong, it will help balance our emotional life.

The best way to see Shen is in its relationship with Qi and Jing. Jing, Qi and Shen are referred to together in Chinese medicine as the "Three treasures". Jing is responsible for developmental activities. Qi is responsible for life and the activity of the body. Shen is the mind or spirit. When the "Three treasures" are harmonious the person will be fit, healthy and mentally alert.[13]

Meridians

In acupuncture Qi moves through the body by a network of channels called meridians. Meridians are invisible channels which link the organs to the rest of the body. Small needles are placed in acupuncture points along the meridians to stimulate the flow of Qi. Acupuncture, acupressure, Tai Chi and Qi Gong help improve the flow of energy or Qi.

In Chinese medicine the organs of the body are systems similar to western medicine but with an energy that includes the meridians.[14] The organ systems or networks are called the Zang Fu Organs.

The Zang Fu System

This is the name for the series of Yin and Yang organ systems in Chinese medicine. The Zang organs consist of the yin organs of lungs, heart, spleen, liver, kidneys and pericardium. The Fu organs are the Yang organs. They are the small intestine, large intestine, gall bladder, stomach, bladder and Sanjiao.[15] The Sanjiao is located separately from the zang fu organs and inside the body. Its meridian connects with the pericardium with which it is externally-internally related.

Zang Fu System:

The Lungs – Zang organ

Lungs govern Inhalation of pure Qi from the air and extraction of impure Qi. It disperses defensive Qi and body fluid and manages the water passages. The Lungs control the skin and hair. The lungs open onto the nose. Grief is the emotion associated with the lungs. They are connected to the Large Intestine Fu organ.

Heart – Zang organ

The heart has the function of transforming Qi from food into blood and the heart houses the mind. The heart controls blood vessels. It is connected to the tongue. The heart is associated with the emotion of joy. It is connected to the small intestine Fu organ.

Spleen – Zang organ

The spleen governs transformation and transportation of foods which depend on spleen Qi. It controls blood. It is connected to the muscles and limbs. It is related to the mouth and lips. It is associated with worry and over-thinking It is related to the stomach Fu organ.

Liver – Zang

Stores blood. It is connected to the ligaments, tendons and nails. It is connected to the eyes. It is related to the emotion of anger. The Fu organ is gallbladder.

Kidneys – Zang

The kidneys dominate reproduction and growth and receive Qi. It also regulates water metabolism. It is connected to the brain and bone marrow. It is associated with the ears. The emotion it is related to is fear, anxiety. The Fu organ is the bladder.

As you can see, each of the Zang organs is linked with a sense organ, a tissue, an emotion and a Fu-organ. For example, the Zang organ of the lungs is connected to the large intestine (Fu organ). The tissue connected with the lungs is the skin and hair. The sense organ connected to the lungs is the nose and the emotion connected to the lungs is grief.[16]

Interconnection of Organs
Each of the organs has a close relationship with the other. How well each organ functions is dependent on how smoothly the blood and Qi move. If the energy flow is blocked in any organ, there will be stagnation. When there is too much Qi, there is excess in the organ, when there is too little Qi, there will be deficiency.

Spleen and kidney network and weight gain
If the spleen becomes damaged by external or internal damp(eg a poor diet), this can result in more dampness that leads to an accumulation of mucus and phlegm.[17] In Chinese medicine, weight gain is the result of four factors; qi deficiency, poor diet, lack of exercise and constitutional factors. Poor diet damages the spleen and stomach network causing dampness and weight gain. Greasy, rich and sweet food increases dampness. Lack of exercise causes poor circulation and stagnation of qi. Stagnation of the fluids in the body can cause dampness and fat. Acupuncture when combined with exercise and a good diet can be very beneficial in weight management.[18]

Balance
Excessive work (which is Yang) will result in deficiency (which is Yin) of the energy of the body. Excessive worrying

(Yang) depletes us. Too much exercise which is (yang) can cause a slow (yin) pulse. Balance in diet, exercise, emotional life and work life is the key to maintaining good health. We should be aware how a Yang condition can change into Yin and how a Yin condition can change into a Yang condition and to avoid extremes of any activity.

If essence and Qi are healthy the mind will be happy and well. A healthy mind is helped by the quality of essence stored in the kidneys and the Qi produced in the spleen and stomach network.

Blood

The primary function of blood is nourishing the body. If blood is deficient, the mind will have no base or foundation and will become uneasy and anxious. When there is blood deficiency we may be more likely to suffer from insomnia.

Wang Ping, a Chinese doctor from the Tang Dynasty said "When the person is active, blood circulates in the vessels, when the person rests, blood goes back to the liver". Sufficient exercise and rest are important for health.[19]

> "The journey of a thousand miles begins with a single step". – Confucius

> "Your teacher can open the door, but you must enter by yourself". – Chinese Proverb

> "Pearls don't lie on the seashore. If you want one, you must dive for it". – Chinese Proverb

CHAPTER FIVE

Acupuncture

Acupuncture derives from ancient Chinese medicine. The basis of present day acupuncture was established during the Ming Dynasty (1368–1644). Acupuncture was first recorded in the ancient Chinese medical text – *The Nei Jing, The Yellow Emperors Classic of Internal Medicine*. Acupuncture has been used in the West since the 17th century.

Acupuncture is a form of Chinese medicine where fine needles are inserted through the skin at acupuncture points. Qi flows through the meridians in the body. The meridians are accessible through the acupuncture points. Inserting fine needles at specific points brings the energy flow into balance.

The World Health Organisation has listed a number of conditions for which acupuncture has been proven effective through controlled trials:

- Allergic rhinitis
- Biliary colic
- Depression
- Dysentery
- Dysmenorrhoea
- Facial pain
- Headache
- Hypertension, essential

- Hypotension, primary
- Knee pain, Low back pain, Neck pain
- Postoperative pain
- Renal colic
- Rheumatoid arthritis
- Bronchial asthma
- Competition Stress Syndrome
- Diabetes mellitus, non-insulin dependent
- Sciatica
- Sprain
- Stroke
- Tennis elbow

Some of the conditions which the World Health Organisation says the therapeutic effect of acupuncture has been shown but for which further proof is needed:

- Bell's palsy
- Female infertility
- Facial spasm
- Female urethral syndrome
- Fibromyalgia
- Gouty arthritis
- Insomnia
- Male sexual dysfunction
- Neuralgia, post-herpetic
- Obesity
- Osteoarthritis
- Polycystic ovary syndrome
- Premenstrual syndrome
- Retention of urine

From The World Health Organisation report – Acupuncture: Review and Analysis of Reports On Controlled Trials – Dr Xiaorui Zhang, World Health Organisation).[1]

Acupuncture treats ill health and excessive weight gain as signs of body imbalance. The goal of acupuncture is to bring the body back into balance. In acupuncture our physical, mental and emotional aspects are regarded as interdependent; reflecting the mind body connection.

Traditional Chinese Medicine treats ill health on the basis that the Qi energy is out of balance in the body and cannot flow freely. This can be caused by stress, poor diet or injury.

What to expect at an acupuncture appointment:
At the first appointment the acupuncturist will take your health history. The acupuncturist may then feel your pulse. Pulse Diagnosis can help the acupuncturist in assessing your condition. Through palpation of the pulse at three locations on both wrists i.e. cun, guan and chi, the general health condition of a person can be established. The ancient Chinese Medical text – *The Nei Jing*, describes over 30 types of pulse e.g. slippery, slow, intermittent etc.

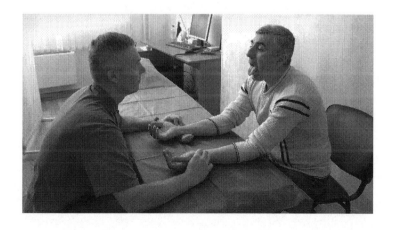

The acupuncturist may then look at your tongue. The tongue has connections to the rest of the body, both to our internal organs and to the meridians(channels). The tongue can give an indicator of a person's general health. The Heart, Spleen, Kidney, Bladder and San Jiao meridians(channels) reach onto the tongue.

The colour of the tongue shows the state of blood, Yin organs and Ying Qi (nutritive Qi). The tongue body shape reflects the state of blood and Ying Qi (nutritive Qi) and indicates Excess or Deficiency. The normal Tongue colour in Traditional Chinese Medicine is pale red.[2]

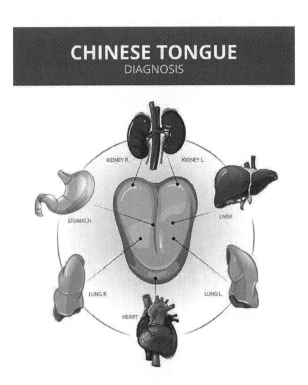

Tongue areas as they correspond to internal organs in Chinese Medicine:

During the acupuncture treatment, the acupuncturist will insert fine sterile disposable needles at specific points throughout the body to improve health on a physical, psychological and emotional level. Most people find acupuncture relaxing and often feel more calm after a treatment. You may feel a little tired afterwards and it is wise to avoid planning vigorous exercise after an acupuncture session.

Many people find when they begin a course of acupuncture treatments that they begin to experience positive changes in their overall health. You may find that you begin to sleep better, feel more relaxed and have a better outlook.

Number of treatments
As every person is unique, the number of treatments required will vary for everyone. Initially you may have one or two treatments a week for about six weeks and you can then space out the treatments. Chronic health conditions take longer to treat than acute conditions and the length of time will depend on the person's overall state of health.

Is acupuncture safe?
Acupuncture is safe and effective when performed by a well-trained practitioner. If you are pregnant or trying for a baby, it is important to let your practitioner know so that the treatment can be modified.

Cupping
Cupping is used in Traditional Chinese Medicine to warm and promote the free flow of qi and blood and to remove stagnation. Cupping involves warming cups and placing them on the skin: by warming the air within the cup, a

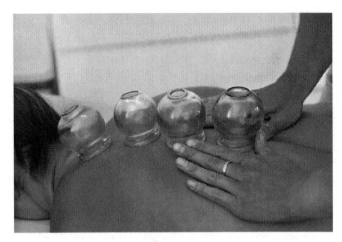

Cupping

vacuum is created and when the cup is applied to the skin, the tissue is drawn up into the cup. This increases blood circulation in the area and is believed to stimulate healing.[3]

Moxibustion
Moxibustion is sometimes used during an acupuncture treatment. It consists of burning moxa, a cone or a stick made of dried mugwort on or near the acupuncture points and meridians. It is used to expel cold and warm the meridians, to help the smooth flow of Qi and blood and to treat deficiency of yin and yang.[4]

Acupuncture and Weight Management
When there is imbalance in the body causing weight gain, it may be caused by liver, spleen, or kidney disharmony, there may also by thyroid or endocrine imbalance.

In one study, acupuncture in combination with diet regulation was found to be effective for weight loss and the reduction of inflammation.[5] Acupuncture is thought to help weight loss by suppressing appetite, boosting the metabolism and reducing stress.

A study published online concluded that acupuncture is a reasonable and effective treatment for people who suffer from obesity. The study also said that hormones including insulin and ghrelin may influence appetite in the hypothalamus.[6]

Combining acupuncture and lifestyle programs for weight management

When using acupuncture while trying to lose weight, best results will be achieved by using the treatment along with healthy lifestyle choices such as healthy diet, exercise and mind body exercise such as meditation, yoga, Tai chi or Qi gong. Acupuncture can help start a healthy lifestyle and weight loss program but the client must also be committed to making changes in their food, exercise, stress levels and sleep habits.

Ear acupuncture

Ear acupuncture is used for many conditions including weight loss. Certain points in the ear can be used to control food cravings. Sometimes an acupuncturist will attach ear seeds to certain points in the ear. The patient can then press the points where the seeds are to stimulate the acupressure points, this helps as a reminder to mindful eating.

Local and distal points

Distal points are located on the limbs. Local points are situated on the trunk and head. A combination of local and distal points is the best way of balancing points.[7]

Eight principle approach

The eight principle approach is used in acupuncture, it is in keeping with the philosophy of Yin and Yang. The eight principles contain four interdependent sets of characteristics: yin and yang, internal and external, cold and hot, deficiency and excess. Every acupuncture treatment is aimed at one of four strategies:

- Tonifying Yang
- Tonifying Yin
- Eliminating excess Yang
- Eliminating excess Yin.[8]

Yin and Yang are always changing and when one is in excess the other is deficient. The aim of Acupuncture is to balance Yin and Yang. There are four types of imbalance:

Excess of yin
An example of this is where there is excess cold (exterior or interior) consuming yang. This is Full-cold.

Excess of yang
An example is excess heat either interior or exterior consuming the body fluids (yin) leading to dryness. This is Full-heat.

Consumption of yang
When the yang energy of the body is not sufficient and is deficient, the lowering of yang energy can cause cold, chilliness and other symptoms. When Yin is weak, Yang is in apparent excess. This is empty- cold.

Consumption of yin
This happens when the yin energy of the body is depleted. When Yang is weak, Yin is in apparent excess. This is empty-heat.

Inter-transformation of yin and yang

Yin and yang although opposite can change into one another. For example excessive activity and work (yang) without proper rest can cause extreme deficiency (yin) of the energy in the body. Excessive exercise (yang) can cause a very slow (yin) pulse. Striving for a state of balance is the key, whether it's in diet, exercise, personal life or work. Frequent swings from yin to yang and vise versa can cause damage to our physical and emotional health.[9]

The six pathogenic factors

The six pathogenic factors can also lead to sickness. They are wind, cold, heat, dampness, dryness and fire. The six factors will only cause damage if the climate changes are severe or if the immune system is low. The six pathogenic factors are related to seasonal changes e.g. heat syndromes usually occur in the summer and cold syndromes in the winter and excessive exposure to damp causes damp syndromes e.g. chest infections and achy joints.[10]

CHAPTER SIX

Acupressure

In acupressure, pressure is applied to key points on the skin to stimulate self-healing. By using these points you stimulate the blood circulation and energy flow (Qi) to help healing.

The same points are used in acupressure and acupuncture. In acupuncture fine needles are used on the points, whereas in acupressure the fingers and hands apply a light pressure to the points. You can use self-acupressure to relieve stress and anxiety.

With the assistance of deep breathing and acupressure you can help improve your health. Acupressure helps inhibit the pain signals to the brain. It can also help balance the body by relieving tension.

The muscle fibres contract when a muscle is in spasm, this is caused by the secretion of lactic acid caused by stress, poor circulation and trauma. The muscle fibres relax and ease when acupressure is applied to a point.

Acupressure has been used as a beauty treatment in China for thousands of years, the use of gentle acupressure helps to improve the condition of the skin and to relax and tone the facial muscles, which helps to stop the appearance of wrinkles.

My first Tai Chi teacher Dr Deng who was also an acupuncturist would always finish the Tai Chi class with a sitting meditation, in which he would get us to gently massage the face in a circular motion, using two fingers on the acupressure points to rejuvenate the face. It probably also explained his youthful complexion.

Local and Distal points
When you stimulate an acupressure point in the area where you feel pain or tension, it is a local point (as in acupuncture). But you can also relieve pain in an area of the body that is distant from the acupressure point (Distal point). This works like a trigger through the meridian channels. The acupressure points are connected to each other through the meridians. The stimulation of one point can send a healing message to other areas of the body.

The Third eye
Some acupressure points can be used for meditation. While using acupressure on the Third Eye point, between the eyes, breathe deeply and meditate for five minutes. This will help to calm the mind when busy or stressed.

Massage Techniques
Massage techniques include using thumbs, fingers, palms or sides of the hands to apply a steady pressure. You can also place the tip of the thumb, index finger or middle finger on the acupressure point and move it in a circle around the point, while applying firm pressure.

Kneading
This motion is like kneading dough; using thumbs, fingers and palms to squeeze areas of the skin.

Effleurage
Effleurage is applied with a soft pressure, it is often used to begin a massage treatment. Effleurage helps blood circulation and uses long strokes.

Quick Tapping
Quick tapping with the fingertips stimulates the muscles on tender areas such as the face.

How to find the right acupressure points
Press gently around the area where the point is supposed to be located. You will find one spot that is more sensitive than the surrounding area. With a little experience you will be able to find a hollow there.

Caution
Do not work directly on infected skin or sore areas. Nor should you work directly on recent scars or after recent surgery. You should not self-treat during pregnancy unless qualified to do so.

If you have an illness which is serious or life threatening such as high blood pressure, heart disease or cancer you should avoid using deep pressure or over-stimulating the acupressure points. Use the abdominal points very cautiously with any serious health conditions and it is strongly advisable to consult a practitioner for treatment.

Anxiety
You can help relieve anxiety by being conscious of your breath. Slow deep breaths help relieve tension. Symptoms of anxiety can include restlessness, exhaustion and insomnia. Panic attacks are also a form of anxiety; if anxiety continues

without treatment, it can weaken our immune system. Where anxiety is chronic you should also consult your G.P.

If you are prone to anxiety you should also get plenty of physical exercise including walking and avoid sugar, caffeine and highly processed food and eat lots of fruit and vegetables. You could also consider the benefits of Tai chi, Qi Gong, meditation or yoga which are wonderful for anxiety.

Bladder 10
This is located one finger width below the base of the skull, a half inch from the spine.

Benefits:
This helps relieve stress, nervousness and anxiety. It also helps muscle discomfort in the neck and shoulder.

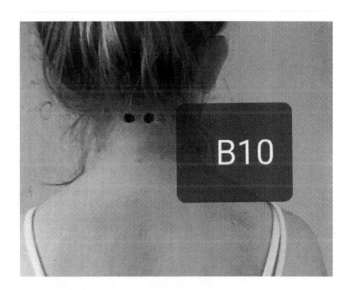

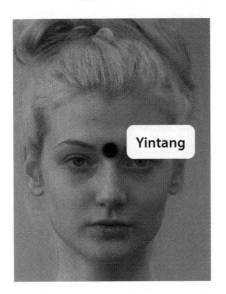

Third eye point (yintang point)
This is located midway between the medial ends of the eyebrows.

Benefits:
Gentle pressure to this point helps relieve nervousness, frontal headache and insomnia.

P6 (Neiguan point)
This is located two fingers widths above the crease of the wrist between the tendons Palmaris longus and flexor radialis.

Benefits:
Gentle pressure helps anxiety, nausea and insomnia.

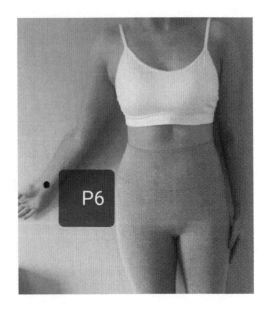

Sea of tranquility (ren 17 point)
This is located midway between the nipples.

Benefits:
Gentle pressure on this point helps relieve anxiety and tension. It is also beneficial for asthma.

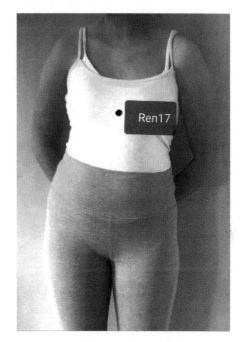

Insomnia

Stress and anxiety can make sleeping disorders worse. Peace of mind is important for falling asleep. Deep breathing and meditation can also help. When we eat a diet high in saturated fat, it may cause elevated cholesterol, this can result in narrowing of the blood vessels. The heart is then forced to work harder to pump the blood, placing the body under stress.

In Chinese medicine, the heart is believed to affect our ability to sleep. Drinking ginger and herbal teas instead of caffeine in the latter half of the day will help calm the body down.

On the Chinese 24 hour Meridian clock (The Circadian Rhythms) if you are awake during the 1am–3am time frame, your liver will not do as good a job on detoxifying your blood. As a result you may not feel rested and be weak at planning and motivation; even if you slept for 8 hours from 3am to 11am! Between 11 pm and 1pm the body builds blood cells and engages in cellular repair more efficiently if we are resting/asleep.

H7
This is located on the inside of the wrist, on the side of the wrist which is in the line of the little finger.

Benefits:
This helps anxiety, cold sweats and insomnia when caused by over-excitement.

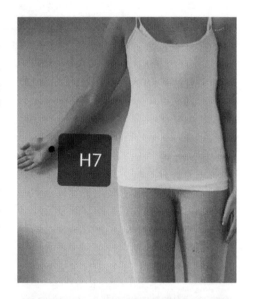

B62
In the depression below the outer ankle.

Benefits:
Insomnia, backache, dizziness.

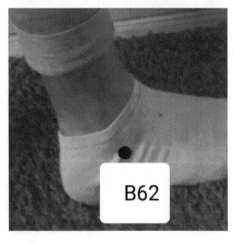

K6
One finger width below the
inside of the ankle.

Benefits:
Insomnia, asthma, retention
of urine.

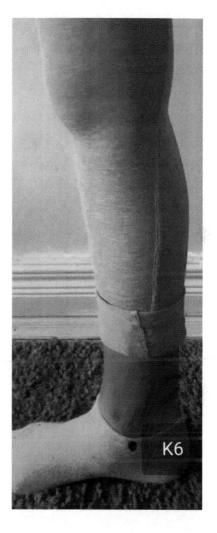

Depression and Emotional balancing

Depression can be a sign that something in our lifestyle is
out of balance. It is important to distinguish between feeling
a little off and more chronic acute depression. For chronic
depression it is necessary to see a G.P.

S36

Three finger widths below the knee, a finger width size to the outside of the shin.

Benefits:
This point helps relieve insomnia, anxiety and indigestion.

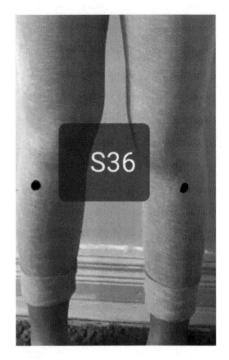

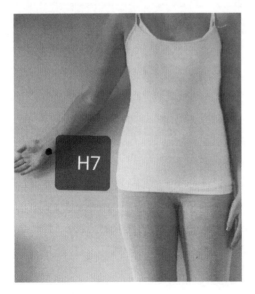

H7
On the little finger side of the hand on the wrist crease.

Benefits:-Depression and Insomnia.

Du 20

On the midline of the head, on the midpoint of the line connecting the apexes of the two ears.

Benefits:
Depression and anxiety.

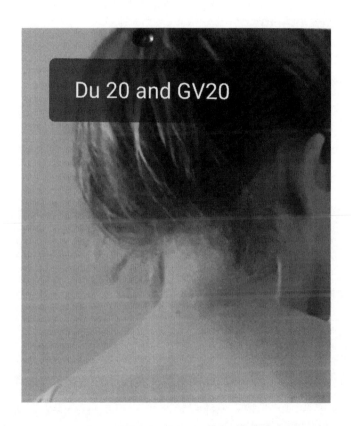

Acupressure and weight loss

It is advisable to make lifestyle changes in the area of diet, exercise, stress and sleep. Mind body exercises in combination with acupressure or acupuncture facilitate weight loss. Acupressure points help weight loss by stimulating the metabolism. When acupressure points are practiced along with relaxation and deep breathing, the acupressure can help curb appetite.

Spleen 6

This is located three finger widths above the inner anklebone.
Benefits:
Helps abdominal distension, oedema and helps boost the metabolism.

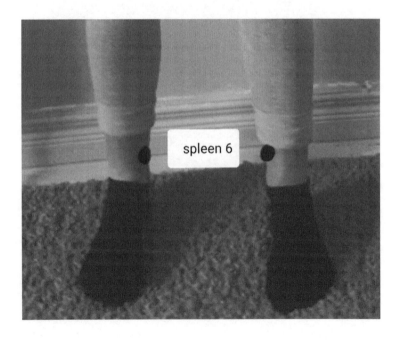

spleen 6

Ren 6
On the midline of the abdomen, one and a half finger widths below the navel.

Benefits:
bloating and constipation

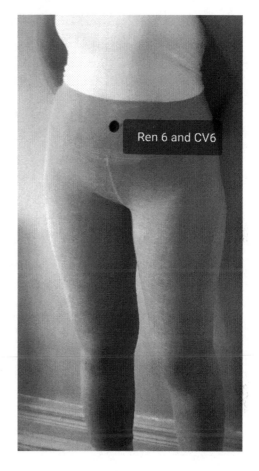

Ren 6 and CV6

CHAPTER Seven

Tai Chi and Qi Gong

"Tai Chi is a natural intervention involving self-motivation and participation, thereby empowering people to manage their own health".

– Andy Choo

Tai chi is an internal Chinese martial art which is practiced for health, fitness and mind body exercise.

The term Tai chi refers to the philosophy of yin and yang. Tai chi originated in China but it is now practiced worldwide. Most styles of Tai chi trace their development to one of the traditional schools which are Chen, Yang, Sun, Wu and Wu (Hao) styles of Tai chi.

The practice of Tai chi strengthens the bones and muscles and regulates the body's energy channels (meridians). There is an old Chinese saying "if plenty of water is feeding the stream, the stream will last longer and go further". If we look after our health, it will pay dividends.

Tai chi is often described as "meditation in motion"; as you move, you breathe deeply and naturally while focusing your attention. In Tai chi and Qi Gong, the Dantian is a point located just three finger widths below your navel, it is the centre store of internal energy and the focal point of the breath. Baihui (Du20) is situated at the top of the head; in

Tai chi, Baihui (Du20) is considered an important point for internal energy flow.

Tai chi consists of still exercises or meditation along with moving exercises called forms. It places equal concentration on body movements and internal energy control. Conscious awareness is practiced with body movements.

By conscious awareness you collect the Qi energy in the body and use it to renew and recharge yourself. During Tai chi practice the Qi energy will concentrate in the Dantian and flow through the body. This will help in emotional balancing and lessens nervousness and anxiety. It also boosts the immune system and is beneficial for health.

By having a relaxed mind during the practice of Tai chi, the energy flow in the body will improve. Regular practitioners of Tai chi will find they have a clearer mind and feel more energised and content.[1]

The ancient Chinese medical text, the *Nei Jing*, puts emphasis on finding interior quiet and clearing the mind when practicing Qi Gong; this is also important for Tai chi.

"As long as the body and spirit remain coherent, longevity can be expected" – *Nei Jing*

"Health and well-being can be achieved, only by remaining centred in spirit, guarding against the squandering of energy, promoting the constant flow of qi and blood, maintaining harmonious balance of yin and yang…and nourishing one's self preventively" – *Nei Jing*

Tai chi, muscle strength and flexibility

Tai chi helps improve upper and lower body strength when practiced regularly. It is comparable to resistance training and brisk walking. Although you are not working with weights or resistance bands, the movements strengthen your upper and lower body. An article from Harvard Health Publishing on Tai Chi says "It also strengthens the lower and upper body extremities, the core muscles and boosts flexibility".[2]

Tai chi for stress reduction

A randomised controlled trial was undertaken to determine whether 12 weeks of Tai chi practice can reduce anxiety in stressed healthy people. It concluded that Tai chi reduces stress levels in healthy individuals and is a safer alternative to some other types of exercise.[3]

Our emotional state has an effect on our breathing. Stress can make us breathe faster. However when we breathe mindfully as in Tai Chi, we will improve relaxation and help our balance. Dr Paul Lam in his book "Teaching Tai Chi effectively" says that when *you* are inhaling and storing energy *you* should "think of taking life energy into your body. When you exhale, think of delivering energy or force".[4]

Tai chi and weight loss

One of the benefits of Tai chi is that you can build muscle which also helps to get rid of excess fat, aiding weight loss. It also improves the metabolism.

A study from the Chinese university of Hong Kong studied the effects of 12 weeks of Tai chi and brisk walking on weight loss and BMD in middle aged Hong Kong adults. It was found that both slightly reduced the body weight and fat mass and had significant improvements on waist circumference.[5]

In the book 'Tai Chi for health' by Grandmaster Chen Zhenglei and Grandmaster Liming Yue it says "one of the benefits of this kind of exercise is its ability to reduce the amount of fat around the muscles and open the pores of your skin, it leaves the skin looking and feeling smoother softer and healthier".[6]

Tai chi can improve cognitive performance and memory in older adults with mild cognitive impairment

A research article from the American society of Neuro-rehabilitation has also shown that Tai chi can improve cognitive performance and memory. The memorisation of a sequence of movements is good exercise for the brain.[7]

Effects of Tai chi compared to aerobic exercise for fibromyalgia

A randomised controlled trial concluded that Tai chi mind body exercise resulted in similar or greater improvement than aerobic exercise for patients with fibromyalgia. The mental and physical aspect of Tai Chi improves fitness and mindset.[8]

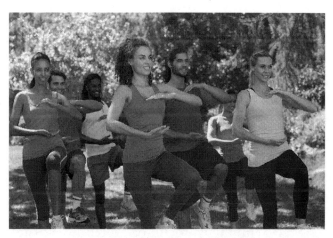

Group Practicing Tai Chi

Qi Gong and Tai chi for mood regulation

Clinical studies have shown that Qi Gong and Tai chi have beneficial effects on psychological well-being and reduce symptoms of anxiety and depression.[9] By focusing on the breath, relaxation and body awareness, we achieve mental quietness and serenity.

Tai chi styles

Chen Style

Chen style Tai chi is the original and oldest form of Tai chi. The Silk reeling exercises and forms incorporate alternating fast and slow motion. Chen Tai chi was created in Chenjiagou village in Henan province China in the late Ming dynasty.

Yang style

The moves in Yang style are slow, gentle and even. Yang style is the most widespread style in the world. The founder of Yang style Tai chi, Yang Luchan, learned the old form of Tai chi from the Chen Grandmaster Chen Changxing.

Sun style Tai chi

This is known for its flowing, smooth movements. Sun style was developed by Sun Lutang. Sun learned Wu (Hao)style from Hao Weizhen.

Wu style Tai Chi

This style uses pushing hands like Chen style, hand forms and horse stance training. The founder of Wu style was a student of Yang Luchan.

Wu (Hao style)

This style is defined by focus on accurate position and internal strength. It was founded by Wu Yuxiang.

Jing

Jing, as distinguished from Jing as essence, is roughly translated as mental quietness or serenity. In the Jing state your mind becomes serene by focusing on body awareness, the breath, and relaxation while loosening the joints. The aim in Tai chi and Qi gong is to attain this Jing state.[10]

> "Using the Jing state will help you to deal with various life crisis. For when a crisis arises you will know how to step back mentally and put yourself in a Jing state from where you can see the situation clearly and deal with it more rationally".   – Dr Paul Lam

Tai Chi and strength training

Tai Chi improves upper and lower body strength and the core muscles but we can supplement it with weight training to maintain muscle strength and to burn fat.

Lifting weights is a very effective way to burn calories. Weight training builds muscle better than cardio (running, walking, cycling, swimming etc). But it is in the resting period after lifting weights that the benefit occurs, helping you to burn off more calories for up to 38 hours afterwards. When you have more muscle, your basal metabolic rate is higher. A study in 2017 which was published in the Journal 'Obesity' reported that adults in their 60's who were overweight, but did strength training and reduced calories, had less muscle loss and significant fat loss compared to calorie reduction plus walking or calorie reduction alone. It is recommended to leave a rest day between strength training for maximum effect. Strength training also helps your bones, reducing your risk of osteoporosis. Consuming protein is also very

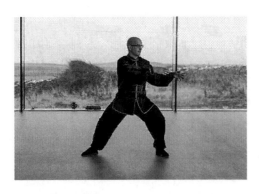

Kevin Copeland, Westway
Tai Chi and Qi Gong

important for building muscle, especially beans, nuts, pulses and a small amount of meat or fish.

We may be inclined to dismiss weight training as a current trend, however in ancient China, just as in Rome and Athens, soldiers practiced weight training to ready themselves for battle. An article in www.physicalculturestudy.com on 'An early history of weightlifting', says that historians have uncovered Chinese documents showing an exercise routine for soldiers. During the period of the Warring states (770 BC to 221 BC) Qiao Guan and Kang Ding were forms of weightlifting that became popular. Records also show weightlifting during the Ming dynasty (1368 to 1644) and the Qing Dynasty (1644 to 1911). In Ancient Egypt a mural from the tomb of Beni Hasan (dating back to about 1650 BC) and other artworks in the tomb, show men and women exercising with weights. We can all learn something from ancient wisdom!

Qi Gong

Qi Gong or Chi gung is a system of coordinated body postures, meditation and breathing which has its roots in Chinese medicine and philosophy. Qi Gong is a practice to cultivate Qi or life force. It is practiced throughout China and the world for relaxation, exercise and self-healing.

The 2013 Chinese Medical Qi Gong textbook says there are many physiological effects of Qi Gong including improvement of cardiovascular and respiratory function.[11] The basis of Qi Gong is cultivating a mindful body by using breathing and exercise. The essence of Qi Gong is energy cultivation. Qi Gong has long been known to be effective in helping to heal illness. The principles on which Qi Gong are based are the same as the rest of Chinese medicine; acupuncture, acupressure, Tai Chi etc. The purpose is to tonify and reinforce depleted Qi, clearing blocked or excess Qi and strengthening internal and external (or defensive Qi). Acupuncture and acupressure can be enhanced by Qi Gong and Tai Chi.[12]

Health benefits of Qi Gong:
1. Improves balance
2. Lowers blood pressure
3. May ease depression
4. Improves sleep
5. Helps digestion
6. Helps balance body temperature
7. Boosts the immune system

There are a number of popular forms of Qi Gong including Five Animals Qi Gong, Six healing sounds, Stick Qi Gong, Ma Wang dui and Ba Duan Jin. Ba Duan Jin is a powerful full body exercise.

The Chinese health Qi Gong association book on Ba Duan Jin says in its preface that "it has been proven that the practice of Ba Duan Jin improves the respiratory system, limb strength, flexibility of the joints and fortifies the nerves, as well as enhances the general balance......It strengthens one's immune system to a degree, and delays the ageing process so as to increase the life span. It also improves one's mental health".[13]

> "Tai chi and Qi Gong exercises have many different methods of practice. Whichever method you choose, the final goal and fundamental purpose is to increase the level of Qi energy within the body and drive it through the 12 main channels (meridians) ... internal energy Qi is the vital living force within every human body".
>
> – Grandmaster Chen Zhenglei and Grandmaster Liming Yue, *Tai chi for health*, published 2005.

Ba Duan Jin is practiced in two positions standing and sitting, but the standing style is more popular. The movements should be flowing and continuous to achieve inner calm and serenity. This helps the circulation of energy and improves health and fitness. Guided by intention and taking a deep breath, the body will relax. The movements which are a mixture of strength and relaxation will help to achieve a balance between Yin and Yang. Ba Duan Jin like other forms of Qi Gong helps to improve circulation in the meridians.

The practice of Ba Duan Jin:
To ensure that you are practicing the routines properly you should attend a Qi Gong class or follow the Chinese Health Qi Gong Association book and also their video on YouTube. Always consult with your G.P. before engaging in any exercise routine.

Routine 1. Holding the Hands high with palms up to help regulate the internal organs.

1. Join the hands, cross the fingers with the palms facing up in front of the stomach. Look straight ahead.
2. Straighten the knees and stand upright. Lifting the hands, with palms upward, then turning the palms inward push the hands skyward, palms up. Raise the head and look at the palms.
3. Straighten the elbows. Pull in the chin and look straight ahead.
4. Bend the knees while lowering the body weight. Hold the hands in a semicircular position in front of the navel with palms up. Look straight ahead.
5. The above movements should be repeated six times.

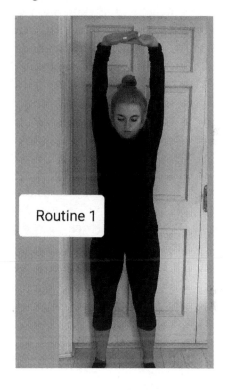

Routine 1

Functions and Benefits:

This routine helps the Sanjiao, which are the three areas housing the internal organs. It assists blood circulation and Qi inside the organs. It also helps shoulder problems and helps prevent neck problems.

Routine 2. Posing as an archer shooting both left and right handed.

1. Stand straight. Raise the hands in front of the chest. Look straight ahead. Separate your feet

2. Slowly bend the knees to the horse stance. Forming a fist with your right hand, move it in front of the right shoulder. Push the left arm out to the left. Bend the left wrist and face the palm left, like an archer preparing to release an arrow. Maintain the position, with eyes looking to the left.

3. Return to centre position with hands in front of chest.

4. Slowly bend knees to horse stance. Forming a fist with left hand, move it in front of left shoulder. Push the right arm to the right. Bend the right wrist and face the palm right, like an archer preparing to release an arrow. Hold the position with the eyes looking to the right.

5. This routine is to be done 6 times. Three times to the left and three times to the right.

6. Finish in centre position, standing straight with feet slightly apart and the knees bent slightly. Move the hands in front of abdomen like holding a ball with the palms up and fingers facing each other. Look straight ahead.

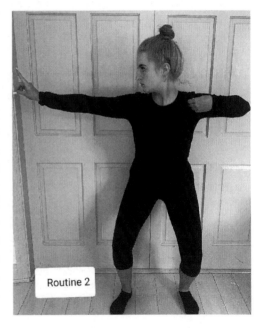

Routine 2

Benefits:

This is good for the Du meridian. It is also good for the lung meridian. It also corrects unhealthy postures.

Routine 3. Holding one arm aloft to regulate the functions of the spleen and stomach.

1. Slowly straighten knees. Raise the left hand to a position above the head on left side with elbow slightly bent. At the same time raise right hand slightly with palms facing down. Hold this position, looking straight ahead.
2. Bring both hands down to a position in front of the abdomen with the palms up. Look straight ahead.
3. Slowly straighten knees. Raise the right hand to a position above the head on the right side with elbow slightly bent. At the same time raise left hand slightly with palms facing down. Hold this position, looking straight ahead.
4. Repeat movements three times to the right side and three times to the left side.
5. Finish by bending knees slightly with palms down to the sides, looking straight ahead.

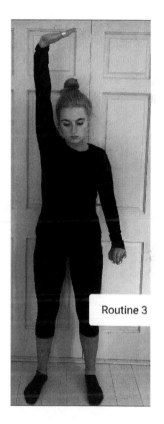

Routine 3

Benefits:

The raising and lowering of the arms has a stretching effect on the abdominal cavity and massages the spleen and stomach organs. This exercise improves the spine's flexibility.

Routine 4. Looking backwards to prevent sickness and strain.

1. Stand with feet apart, with hands to the sides, with hands slightly out and palms facing back. Look straight ahead. Turn the arms outward with palms facing back. Turn the head left to the back. Pause, looking back to the left.
2. Come back to centre position. Turn the arms inward, press the palms down to the sides.
3. Move hands slightly out and palms facing back. Look straight ahead. Turn the arms outward with palms facing back. Turn the head right to the back. Pause, looking back to the right.
4. Repeat routine three times to the left and three times to the right.
5. Finish by moving the hands to a position in front of abdomen, palms up, looking straight ahead.

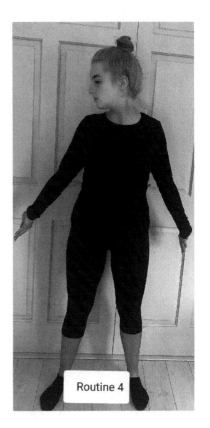

Routine 4

Benefits:

This routine is good for disorders related to the heart, liver, spleen, lungs and kidneys as well as stress from anger, grief, worry and fear. It improves the movements of the neck and shoulder muscles.

Routine 5. Swinging the head and lowering the body to relieve stress.

1. Raise the hands and turn the arms inward when they are chest high. Continue lifting the hands above the head, with elbows slightly bent, palms up and fingers pointing to each other. Look straight ahead.
2. Slowly bend the knees to assume a horse stance. Place hands on thighs. Look straight ahead.
3. Move body weight to the right.
3. Move the head and body in a circular motion to the left.
4. Shift the body weight to horse stance, with hands on thighs.
5. Repeat movements three times to the left and three times to the right.

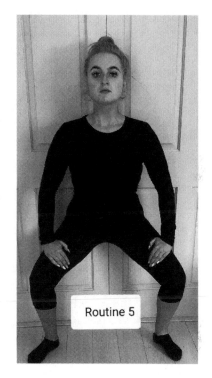

Routine 5

6. Finally stand feet shoulder width apart. Raise hands to above the head. Bring the arms down with hands pointing to each other. Look straight ahead.

Benefits:
This is good for the Du meridian. It helps regulate the inner energy circulation to get rid of stress. The swing helps flexibility.

Routine 6. Moving the hands down the back and legs, and touching the feet to strengthen the kidneys.

1. In standing position, straighten the knees, with the feet apart. Raise the arms over the head and the palms facing forward. Look straight ahead.
2. Turn the arms to face palms. Press the hands down to the front of the chest with palms down and fingers pointing to each other.
3. Move the hands to the back of the upper body from under the armpits.
4. Move the hands along the sides of the spine and to the hips and tilt the upper body forward. Move the hands down along the backs of the thighs and to the insteps past the arches of the feet. Raise the head and maintain this position for a while.
5. Move the palms forward along the floor, then raise the arms and upper body with elbows straight and palms facing forward.

Routine 6

6. Repeat six times. Then bend knees slightly and bring hands to a position in front of abdomen with palms facing down.

Benefits:
Good for the spine and Du meridian. Helps urogenital system by strengthening the kidneys and waist.

Routine 7. Thrusting the Fists and Making the Eyes Glare to enhance Strength.

1. Move the body weight to the right. Move the left foot to the left one step to adopt a horse stance. Clench the fists at the sides of the waist.
2. Slowly thrust the clenched fist forward to shoulder level. Make the eyes glare while looking at the left fist.
3. Turn the left arm inward. Look at the left palm. Turn the left arm outward, elbow slightly bent. Look at the left fist.
4. Bend the left elbow to withdraw the fist to the side of the waist. Look straight ahead.
5. Repeat movements three times to the left and three times to the right. Then move the body weight to the right and withdraw the left foot to stand straight with the feet together. Unclench the fists and let the arms hang loose, looking straight ahead.

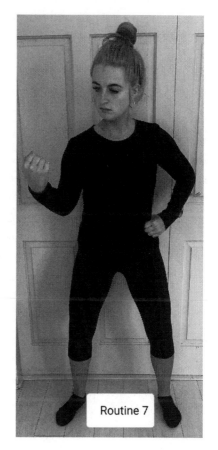

Routine 7

Benefits:

In traditional Chinese medicine, the liver is linked to the tendons and sinews and is connected to the eyes. By making the eyes glare, it stimulates the liver channel and helps improve blood circulation.

Routine 8. Raising and Lowering the Heels.

1. Standing straight, raise the heels. Pause and look straight ahead.
2. Lower the heels to tap them lightly on the floor, looking straight ahead.
3. Repeat movements seven times.

Benefits:

This routine can stimulate the channels and collaterals of the feet and regulate the functions of the related organs. Tapping the heels stimulates the spine and meridians and improves blood circulation.[14]

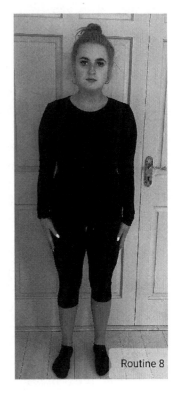

Routine 8

CHAPTER EIGHT

Meditation

....

"The aim of meditation is to train our mind towards intuitive wisdom. When meditating try to think of nothing and let your mind go free".
                                        – Adeline Yen Mah

We can fritter so much time and energy in constant activity distracted from ourselves. Meditation brings us back to our self. Meditating is like taking a break from our overcrowded minds to an oasis which is calm and care free. A Tai Chi Master I attended for training workshops would meditate during breaks to improve focus and attention. I was fascinated that he could contentedly sit and meditate with some light food to enhance his concentration, while we the students headed off for a full lunch!

In our local community centre where I live in Tipperary, Ireland, my two friends Helen and Maura and I have led a community meditation group for the last eight years. Some of the people coming to our group have meditated for many years and we learn much from their wisdom. We all learn from each other and have benefited hugely from the enthusiasm and motivation within the group.

If we can train the mind we can achieve anything. If we set aside time to discipline our minds to meditate we will achieve greater clarity. We can start with ten to twenty minute time blocks, the first block when we wake up in the morning. The more committed you are to your meditation practice, the more the relaxed focus will infuse your day.

In the stillness of meditation, we can reconnect with our inner core which we may have lost connection with through constant rushing and busyness. The practice of mindfulness in the Buddhist tradition is called Calm Abiding. It brings all the parts of ourselves which have been distracted to a place of inner peace. It also helps us to be more positive. Instead of suppressing our emotions we can acknowledge and deal with them. We can learn to be "etre bien dans sa peau" (comfortable in our own skin) as native French speakers would say.

Anyone who meditates regularly will be aware of its relaxing effect on the body and mind. Your capacity in coping with stressful situations improves, you have more energy and focus. By being more relaxed, we can find it easier to prioritise what is really important.

In the book "The Relaxation Response" by Dr Herbert Benson, Dr Benson says traditional methods of meditation can create the relaxation response. He says they will be effective as long as there is 1) A quiet environment 2) An object for the attention to dwell on 3) A passive attitude 4) A comfortable posture such as sitting.[1]

The Three Tools of Meditation

There are Three Tools that are effective in meditation. They are 1) Resting on an object. 2) Observing the breath. 3) Using a mantra.

1) Resting on an object. Here you fix your mind lightly on an object. It could be a picture of anything that has meaning

for you. This may be a candle, it may be a picture. It is what your attention can turn on and rest. Our attention will wander but the meditation object is something to come back to time after time. In meditation our attention and awareness work together. In Yoga meditation "dhyana" is meditation or contemplation when attention becomes awareness.

2) Observing the breath. This is resting your mind and your attention mindfully on the breath. Every time you breathe out and before inhaling there will be a space. When you breathe in, do not place your attention on the in breath, just focus on the in-between space, do not delay your in breath or exhalation. Breathe gently and deeply into the abdomen. As you become more mindful of your breathing you will become more centred. When you start your practice spend the first two to three minutes in passive observation of your breathing. This will calm the mind more quickly. The Japanese call the point a couple of finger widths below the navel 'the tanden' as the focus point for breathing. This is also called the Dantian.

3) Reciting a mantra. Your mantra can be any word you choose. It could be as simple as the word "peace" or the word "OM" (which signifies the essence of the ultimate reality or consciousness.) The "OM" sound is primordial sound. You can also use the mantra "Maranatha" an Aramaic phrase which means Come Lord. By reciting the mantra quietly, just allow your breath, the mantra and your awareness become one.

Basic technique:
1. Meditate in a quiet place free from distractions.
2. Sit relaxed and comfortable.

3. Breathe quietly, gently, smoothly in rhythm. Breathe through the nostrils and down into the abdomen.
4. Let your attention focus on your breathing. You should breathe into the lower abdomen. The lower abdomen is the focus of awareness.
5. Count your exhalation of breath from one to five.
6. Observe a relaxed passive attitude towards distractions, every time you become aware that your mind is wandering, become mindful of your breathing and restart with.... one...two etc.

Awareness of breathing is practiced in the Buddhist tradition in India, Tibet, Japan, China and across South East Asia. The tradition of breathing meditation is associated with peace of mind and improving mental and physical health.

When we are calm, we breathe slowly and smoothly. When we are stressed, we hold our breath. There is a connection between our breath and our emotional life. Awareness of quiet abdominal breathing calms and stabilises the nervous

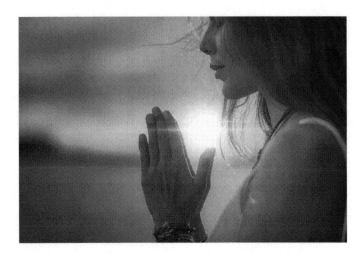

system and improves muscular and mental relaxation. We can last for a few days without food or water, but only a few minutes without air. Breathing is under the control of the voluntary and involuntary nervous systems. We have been given the ability to slow and speed up our breathing, to sing and to hold our breath to try to stop breathing harmful fumes. The Yogis use breath control as central to practice.[2]

Distractions
When practicing meditation, keep returning your mind to the breath. This will gradually calm the mind. Whenever thoughts and emotions arise let them go, just like the ocean waves. Your approach to distractions should be passive. As soon as you become aware of the distraction gently and without irritation bring your attention back to the object. Chogyam Trungpa a Tibetan Buddhist said in relation to distractions that "one should not try to suppress thoughts in meditation, but one should try to see the transitory nature, the translucent nature of thoughts". The point of meditation is to develop acceptance of everything including distractions. When you meditate regularly, the periods of non distraction become more prolonged.

In Lu K'uan Yu's book 'The secrets of Chinese Meditation' he discusses the extent to which the Chinese have practiced awareness of breathing both for better health and mystical contemplation.[3]

Where to Meditate
A quiet spot where you live is the best place to meditate regularly, setting out a cushion and maybe a candle will help you to build a routine around meditation. Closing the eyes will also help to shut out distractions. Patanjali the

'Father of Yoga' said closing the eyes is pratyahara or "sense withdrawal". Katsuki Sekida in his book 'Zen Training' instructs that the eyes should be closed during meditation.[4]

Posture

The easiest posture is the cross legged position. The ankles are crossed and the knees are kept as low as possible. The back is upright and the hands are cupped in the lap. The Eastern cross legged position has long been associated with the practice of meditation. The Eastern sages believed that the poise of body enhanced poise of mind.

How long should I meditate?

Twenty minutes is a good time to reach a satisfactory state of meditation. If you are deeply stressed you may need a little longer. After meditating for approximately twenty minutes early in the day; it is a good idea to take mini meditation breaks of about five minutes throughout the day to prolong the benefits.

> "If this elephant of mind is bound on all sides by the cord of mindfulness, all fear disappears and complete happiness comes". – Shantideva

Practicing Mindfulness

> "The best way to capture moments is to pay attention. This is how we cultivate mindfulness. Mindfulness means being awake". – Jon Kabat Zinn

Research from brain scans shows that people who spend their days rushing and finding it difficult to be in the moment, have an amygdala that is on high alert all the time. When we think of other concerns as well as the present one, our bodies' fight or flight system does not switch off. When we become more mindful, we bring our intentions and our actions back into alignment, instead of going into autopilot.[5]

The Four Applications of Mindfulness are set out in The Buddha's 'Satipatthana Sutta'. They are:

1. Awareness of the body
2. Awareness of the feelings
3. Awareness of states of mind
4. Awareness of the contents of the mind.

Awareness begins with mindfulness of breathing. In Satipatthana Sutta it says "a monk...having gone to the forest, to the foot of a tree, or to an empty place, sits down cross-legged, keeps his body erect and his mindfulness alert. Just mindful he breathes in and mindful he breathes out". Mindfulness has been a buzz word in recent years but the term has been used since antiquity!

In practicing mindfulness we must also practice self-compassion. When we are stressed and our thinking is in the past or the future, remember to breathe in the present, the breath is the present. We need to be managers of our thoughts and energy.

Indian Yoga and Chinese Taoism practiced "watching the breath" to let go and let it become a focal point of awareness.

> "When we define ourselves by who we are instead of by what we do, our focus is on achieving inner qualities like serenity, strength, balance, passion or insight".
> – Ingrid Bacci – *The Art of Effortless living*

Calm Meditation

In achieving a state of tranquillity, you can make life easier and reap the health benefits.

Sitting down, drop the shoulders, but keep the back upright, place your palms on your knees. Take a deep breath and practice conscious breathing. Turn the mind within. Say to yourself –

> "I am not the body nor the mind nor the feelings. I am neither sight nor speech nor hearing nor taste. I am not the five senses. The body is the outer covering of the self which is pure and perfect. I am the boundless, the limitless, the deathless spirit. I am the ever free. I am the eternal present. I am who I am". – Selvarajan Yesudian

By repeating this you will train and discipline your mind to a state of calmness. It is beneficial to repeat this for twenty minutes if possible. Meditation helps us to choose what is important.

> "In a conflict between the head and the heart, choose the heart". – Vivekananda

Relaxation Exercise

I am relaxing the muscles at the top of my head
I am relaxing the muscles of my face
I am now beginning to relax
I relax the muscles of my neck and shoulders
I am now beginning to feel relaxed and calm
I am relaxing the muscles down my back
I am becoming more relaxed and calm
I relax the muscles in my arms and hands
I relax the muscles in my legs
I am becoming calmer and more relaxed
My body is calm, I am peaceful.

In her book 'Understanding Meditation' Naomi Humphrey says "Meditation is a conscious act. It might be thought of as the creation of a personal inner sanctuary to which you are able to retreat. Meditation involves deep physical relaxation and the creation of a quite different mental state. It allows you to step outside the pressures of work, home, and relationships. For a short time you are able to leave the worries of the daily round elsewhere".[6]

Eating Mindfully

"Eating a meal in mindfulness is an important practice" says Thich Nhat Hanh. In his book 'Peace in every step' he says we should see that eating a meal is an exercise in mindfulness and that we should see sitting down to eat as a ritual. He advises that when everyone is seated and the food is on the table, we should breathe and say: "Breathing in, I calm my body. Breathing out, I smile", three times. He goes on to say "We can recover ourselves completely after three breaths like this".[7]

Sometimes, if I am driving on the motorway, I will pull into the service station for a cup of tea in the fast food restaurant there. I often notice that there are two kinds of approaches to eating. Some people are savouring each bite and seem to be fully mindful of what they are eating, the second group are totally distracted by their phones while eating, and seem to be barely conscious of what they are putting in their mouths. Savouring your food mindfully is important for the digestive system.

The Raison meditation is an excellent way to learn mindful eating. It is described in the book 'Mindfulness' by Mark Williams and Danny Penman. You get a few raisins, then taking one of the raisins you hold it in your palm; you look at it mindfully, feeling the weight, observing it. Examine every part of it. You then turn the raisin over and continue to explore it. Observing the raisin, notice does it have a scent? Then slowly place the raisin in your mouth. Feel the sensations of it on your tongue without chewing. Savour it in your mouth. Then start to slowly chew the raisin, noticing the taste, slowly chew without swallowing. Then, swallowing the raisin, notice the sensations of swallowing. After you have swallowed the raisin, notice if there is an aftertaste and what the experience felt like.

Loving kindness meditation

Metta or loving kindness meditation is a method to develop compassion for ourselves and others. Loving kindness is unconditional, it does not matter whether we think we "deserve it" or not. We begin by loving and having compassion for ourselves, if we don't have acceptance for ourselves it is hard to extend it to others.

To start, sit down and relax. Focus on the chest area, your heart centre. Breathe in and out, anchor your thoughts and recite to yourself...

"May I be well,
May I be safe and protected,
May I be happy,
May I be healthy and strong,
May I be free of mental suffering".

Then after a couple of weeks you will be ready to also recite the metta for others e.g. may he/she be well...etc. Let the compassion spread through your whole body, mind and heart.

Self-compassion can help lower the stress hormone cortisol

and it also helps to improve the immune system. Dr Patrizia Collard in her book 'Journey into mindfulness' says that:

"Self compassion can be seen as the yin to mindfulness
– the yang".[8]

"My religion is kindness". – The Dalai Lama

Meditation and Health

Studies have shown that meditation can have a positive effect on our health. A study that was funded by the US National Institute of Health discovered that Transcendental Meditation leads to a large reduction in mortality. There was a 30 percent decrease in the rate of cardiovascular mortality and a 49 per cent decrease in the rate of mortality due to cancer in the meditation group compared to the combined controls.[9]

Professor Marie Asberg from the Karolinska Institute in Stockholm is an expert in the area of burnout. She describes the Exhaustion Funnel as an example how this can happen to us. The top of the Funnel is how we are when we are living a balanced life, but as life gets busier, the funnel narrows as we give up things to focus on what seems important. As the stress continues we give up more and more and the circle narrows even more. You are eventually shot out at the bottom, a stressed out shadow of your former self.[10]

You may then have wreaked havoc on your immune system, leaving you open to Chronic Fatigue, Fibromyalgia and other diseases.

"Be strong, and enter into your own body; for there your foothold is firm. Consider it well, O my heart! Go not elsewhere, Put all imaginations away, and stand fast in that which you are". – Kabir

CHAPTER NINE

The Lungs

"The Lungs are like a Minister from whom policies are issued". – *The Yellow Emperors Classic*

Taking care of our lungs and immunity has never been more important especially with the rise in coronaviruses.

Coronaviruses are a family of viruses ranging from the common cold to MERS, SARS and COVID-19. In Chinese medicine, the lung is a yin organ.

Functions of the Lungs

1) Our lungs govern respiration and Qi.

When the function of the lung in dominating the Qi is normal, respiration is smooth. A deficiency of Lung Qi can lead to shortness of breath, fatigue and feeble speech. The lungs govern the overall Qi in the body. The lungs take in oxygen and expel carbon dioxide.

2) They also influence the skin and hair.

The lungs obtain fluids from the spleen and distribute them to the skin. This nourishes and moisturises the skin and hair. When Lung Qi is strong, there will be good resistance to attack by external pathogenic factors e.g. viruses, infections. When Lung Qi is not strong, defensive Qi will also be weak and there may increased perspiration.

3) The Qi of the Lungs help control blood circulation.
The Lungs control circulation in the blood vessels and in the channels. When Lung Qi is strong, the circulation of Blood and Qi will be good and the limbs will be warm.

4) They regulate water passages.
If this function is not normal, there may be fluid retention and oedema. When this function is normal, urination will be normal, when it is impaired there may be urinary retention.

5) They control descending and dispersing.
Dispersing means distributing. The defensive Qi and body fluid is distributed to the whole body to warm and moisten the muscles, skin and hair. The harmony of the lungs will tell if defensive Qi is strong enough to protect the body from viruses and infections. Lung Qi descends to promote the circulation of Qi. Dysfunction in descending can lead to upward movement of Qi and shortness of breath, cough and stuffiness in the chest.

6) They open into the nose.
The nose is the starting point of respiration. Our sense of smell depends on Lung Qi. Some people who have been infected with coronaviruses have noted a loss of their sense of smell.

7) They house the Corporeal Soul.
The Lungs are the home of the Corporeal Soul. The Corporeal soul is affected by the emotions of sadness or grief. These emotions have an effect on breathing. The acupuncture and acupressure point LU-7 has a releasing influence on unexpressed emotions and BL-42 tonifies Lung Qi.[1]

"The Lungs are the root of Qi, the residence of the Corporeal Soul(Po), they manifest in the hair, they fill up the skin, they represent yin within the yang."
– *The Yellow Emperors Classic*

It is very important to pay attention to strengthening the lungs to boost immunity. Regular exercise such as walking, Qi Gong, Tai Chi or Yoga will improve the circulation of Qi.

The lungs are a Zang organ and the Fu organ that the lungs are linked with is the large intestine. According to Chinese medicine the body's immunity and defensive energy is dependent on the strength of the lung and the colon.

Lung patterns may be excess or deficient. Deficiency of Qi is the most important Deficiency pattern of the lungs. Most of the excess patterns arise from invasion of the lungs from external pathogenic factors e.g. infections and viruses. The Qi of the body can be weak due to overwork, bad diet and emotional stress.[2]

Diet
Too much cold foods e.g. dairy and raw foods (warm salads are preferable in the middle of winter) cause dampness which affects the spleen and causes phlegm. Fermented foods also help your digestion and your lungs.

Beneficial foods for the lungs include:
Garlic, sweet potato, ginger, almonds, apples, oats, sesame seeds and leafy green vegetables.

Lung Cleanse Tea Recipe:
1 cup coconut milk heated
2 inches ginger root cut into small pieces

one quarter tsp of turmeric powder
pinch of ground black pepper
1 tsp local honey
Pinch of ground cinnamon

Emotions
Grief and worry are associated with the lungs. Chronic grief and worry over a prolonged period cause lung Qi deficiency and stagnation of Qi. Looking after our emotional health is important in Chinese medicine. Take some paper and pen and write a long letter to yourself expressing your fears, worries, grief, frustrations and anxieties. When you have finished writing it, carefully digest it and examine ways you could change your priorities to live a more self- fulfilled life. This is an exercise in self-awareness.

Lifestyle
A sedentary lifestyle and lack of exercise weakens lung Qi. Physical exercise such as walking, swimming and gym work are good for the lungs. Qi Gong exercises such as Ba Duan Jin and the Healing sounds are particularly beneficial for the lungs.

Tips for lung health:
1. Let go of items you no longer need. Getting rid of old unused clothes, books, furniture etc gives you more head and breathing space. Healthy lung Qi is associated with good communication and clear thinking.
2. Keep warm especially in cold weather. You can save lung energy by keeping warm.
3. Drink warming soups and ginger tea in cold weather. Warm stews and casseroles are also good.

4. Be kind to yourself. The lungs thrive on positive emotions and respect. Valuing yourself shows respect for yourself and you are more likely to attract respect from others, this will also help your lung energy.

Herbs that are beneficial for the lungs
Ginseng Root
Ginseng is nourishing for the lungs, skin and stomach.

Astragalus
It is one of the most common Chinese herbs for strengthening immunity. It is good for chest conditions. Consult with your G.P. before taking this.

Cordyceps mushroom
This is good for lung strength and immunity. It is also helpful in resisting bacteria and viruses. Consult with your G.P. before taking this.[3]

Acupuncture and Acupressure
Both Acupuncture and acupressure are beneficial for lung health. Acupuncture and acupressure will help the body to re-balance and help with healing emotional blockages in the body.

CHAPTER TEN

Herbs and Supplements

If you intend trying any of the herbs and supplements outlined in this chapter, you must check with your doctor or pharmacist beforehand that they do not interact with any medication that you are already taking and that they are suitable for you.

Even if we try to maintain a balanced diet, there are many herbs and supplements that may help to balance, regulate and nourish the body especially if we are deficient in certain minerals or vitamins. There is no 'one size fits all', one herb or supplement may not be required by one individual but may help another.

If you find that any herb/supplement is not suiting you, you should discontinue use immediately.

Cinnamon – This spice has been prized for its properties for thousands of years. The oily part of cinnamon is high in a compound called cinnamaldehyde. Scientists believe this compound has a powerful effect on our health and metabolism. It is an antioxidant and anti-inflammatory.

Citrus Peel – Citrus peel contains beneficial compounds such as d-limonene, terpinolene and citral which help balance blood sugar and liver detoxification. Lemon peel is high in antioxidants. Sip warm water with citrus slices or peel throughout the day.

Dandelion – Dandelion can be eaten cooked or raw. It is often dried and consumed as a tea. Dandelion is full of potent antioxidants. Chicoric and chlorogenic acid are two compounds in dandelion. They may reduce blood sugar. Animal studies showed that dandelion has a protective effect on liver disease.[1]

Milk Thistle – The ingredients in milk thistle are a group of compounds known as silymarin. The silymarin from milk thistle has antioxidant and anti-inflammatory properties. A recent study found that people routinely taking silymarin had a reduction in their fasting blood sugar levels.[2]

Seaweed – Seaweed are forms of algae from the sea. Seaweed is most commonly eaten in Asian countries like Japan, Korea and China. It can be used in soups, stews, sushi rolls, salads and smoothies. The thyroid relies on iodine to make hormones. When you have insufficient iodine you could start to experience weight changes, fatigue or swelling of the neck over time.

Seaweed has the ability to absorb concentrated amounts of iodine from the ocean. Nori seaweed has 25% of the RDI of iodine, Wakame seaweed has approximately 93% of the RDI, Kombu seaweed has 1,682% of the RDI. Kelp is a great source of iodine. The protein present in spirulina and chlorella contain all the essential amino acids. Sugars found in seaweed which are called sulphated polysaccharides can increase the growth of "good" gut bacteria. Seaweed is also thought to have anti-obesity effects. A number of animal studies suggest that fucoxanthin in seaweed may help reduce body fat. A study in Japan revealed that fucoxanthin which is a substance in brown seaweed could help improve blood sugar control.[3]

Turmeric – Curcumin is the main ingredient in turmeric. It has powerful anti-inflammatory properties and is a strong antioxidant. Curcurmin is not easily absorbed into the bloodstream. It helps to take black pepper with it. Curcurmin is fat soluble so it could be a good idea to take it with a little fat. Some studies have noted that curcumin helps arthritis.[4]

Astragalus – Astragalus is a large genus of the legume family Fabaceae. The plant is a perennial that is native to regions of the Northern Hemisphere. It is seen as an adaptogen that helps restore metabolic balance after stressful situations. It is a tonic for the circulation and it helps the immune system.

Ginkgo Biloba – This herb helps improve blood and oxygen flow to the brain and is helpful in treating dementia, anxiety and concentration.

Chinese Yam – This is a vine that is native to Asia. Chinese yam is mainly used for the stomach and spleen, but is also thought to help the kidneys and lungs in Chinese medicine. It has also been found to be rich in DHEA, which is the mother hormone to oestrogen, progesterone and testosterone. It may also help to stabilise blood sugar.

Dong Quai – This has been used in women's health for thousands of years throughout China and Asia. It may regulate menstrual periods and is also used to relieve hot

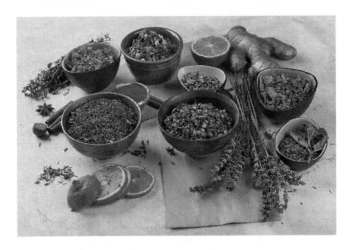

flashes and other menopausal symptoms. It can also help with the immune system.

Ginseng (Panax Ginseng) – This is an energy tonic and has been used for thousands of years for physical and mental endurance. It has been used to help with physical performance. Studies have confirmed that it helps with blood circulation and that it helps prevent heart disease.

Valerian – Valerian has been used for centuries as a herbal remedy. It is used to relieve tension, irritability, stress, anxiety and insomnia.[5]

Supplements – Co Enzyme Q10 – This supplement boosts energy and stamina. It helps with exercise performance. It also helps to regulate blood sugar levels. CoQ10 may protect cells from oxidative stress and helps cellular energy production.[6]

Selenium – It acts as a powerful antioxidant. It is good for heart health and it boosts the immune system.

Vitamin E –This is an antioxidant. It also helps the immune system.

Vitamin C – is needed for the manufacture of collagen in the body and helps the immune system.

Chromium – helps regulate blood sugar and is used for hypoglycemia.

L-Carnitine – It helps to burn fat and may help in weight loss.

Melatonin – It is often used as a sleep aid to help insomnia.[7]

CHAPTER ELEVEN

Visualisation and Goals

If you want to achieve something, you have to visualise it first. Take a comfortable seat. Fix an image in your head of what you want to achieve in health terms, hold that image. Now, taking a deep breath, see yourself in a movie screen on the wall ahead. See yourself eating healthily and doing your mind body and fitness exercises. Imagine for yourself how you feel to be taking care of your body, how good you feel about yourself, really feel the emotion. Say out loud "I now make time for eating and exercising healthily – I make time for me".

This may involve setting new boundaries with the people in your life. But if you don't establish boundaries, you won't have a proper sense of self. Make an appointment with yourself daily to go through this exercise, visualising your new healthy self. You will be engaging your subconscious mind in making the changes to achieve the new healthy lifestyle that you have visualised. The daily repetition of this exercise, visualising your success, will reinforce your goals and will hasten your desired outcome.

Your subconscious mind is in control of over 90% of your actions. Your subconscious is in charge of your behaviour, so if you want changes we have to bring it on board. Creating an image board for yourself will help to engage your subconscious. Cut out pictures of physical exercise and put a picture, any picture, of yourself beside it, also do the same with pictures of healthy food and mind body exercise, placing any pictures of yourself beside the other pictures. Your mind will begin to associate with the new behaviours and you will be assisting your subconscious mind in changing your behaviour.

Writing your goals also helps, write down your new health goals physical and mental. Bring your written goals and some pictures, quotations etc in a journal with you wherever you go and take them out when stuck in traffic or when you have a minute. Visualise and see yourself as successful.

You can also listen to podcasts and audio on healthy living to reinforce your positive changes. The more you engage in visualisation, in all of the forms above, the more you will start believing your goal is possible. We get what we expect. High Performance athletes use mental rehearsal and visualisation to reach their goal.[1]

> "What the mind can conceive and believe, the mind can achieve. Because you visualise your intended destination, your subconscious mind is affected by this self-suggestion. It goes to work to help you get there".
>
> Napolean Hill and W. Clement Stone
> *(Success through a positive mental attitude).*[2]

In his book 'Infinite possibilities' Mike Dooley outlines the principle **"Thoughts become things, is the be all and end all of how to live the life of your dreams"**. He recommends 1) Not visualising for more than 5 minutes each time and the results will prevail over day to day worrying. 2) Be easy with yourself and don't beat yourself up, if your mind strays at the beginning. 3) Feel the emotion when visualising. Feel the joy and happiness associated with the image. 4) Not to visualise for more than five minutes twice daily or the effects will be diluted.[3]

Autosuggestion

I have already mentioned in an earlier chapter Emile Coue, the French psychologist who created the Coue method. He believed that fixing some of our problems requires a change in our unconscious thought, which can be obtained by using the imagination. Initially he used hypnosis but then started using autosuggestion and observed that his patients could cure themselves, by replacing old thoughts with new ones. He believed that repeating images or words helps the subconscious to take them in.[4]

> "Conscious autosuggestion is based on this principle-every idea that we have in our mind becomes true for us and tends to realize itself".   – Emile Coue

In his book 'Self Mastery through Conscious Autosuggestion' Coue says "Every morning before you get up and every evening as soon as you are in bed, shut your eyes, and repeat twenty times in succession 'day by day in every way I am getting better and better'. Do not think of anything in particular, as the words 'in every way' apply to everything. Make this autosuggestion with confidence, with faith, with the certainty of obtaining what you want. The greater the conviction, the greater and more rapid will be the results obtained".

Willpower

Willpower alone is not enough to make changes. Willpower comes from the conscious mind. It is the subconscious that makes the conscious mind do what it wants. When you engage both the conscious and subconscious you will have the willpower. Unhealthy eating and exercise habits have their origins in the subconscious, you have to change this to start living a new healthy lifestyle.

Self-suggestion has an influence on our willpower. Repeat to yourself a number of times in succession 'I am doing what I resolved to do, I am successful in my health goals'. Visualise your self-suggestions. See yourself as healthy, eating the right food and taking your exercise.

> Instil enthusiasm into your will, through reflection and self suggestion. Compel yourself to make progressive efforts... You will soon be conscious of progress, and this will stimulate your zeal and guarantee final success.
> – Raymand de Saint-Laurent

Self-Hypnosis

The use of hypnosis for healing was first recorded in the Middle East over 5000 years ago in ancient Egypt. Self-hypnosis is a self-induced state of hypnosis. It is frequently used alongside self-suggestion or autosuggestion and visualisation to enhance results.

It is easier to access the subconscious mind when relaxed. Sit in a comfortable position. Start taking deep breaths and close your eyes. Say to yourself 'I am going into a state of relaxation. My mind, my body are slowly relaxing. I am going deeper into a state of relaxation. Every muscle in my body is now relaxing. My neck and shoulders are now relaxing. My back is releasing and relaxing. My stomach area is relaxing and now my legs. I am going deeper and deeper into relaxation'. You can go through the exercise again until you are sufficiently relaxed.

Now select one or two affirmations and repeat each affirmation up to 20 times. At the same time visualise your result. When you are finished with the exercise, repeat to yourself. 'I am now coming out of this relaxed state, on the count of three....One, I am totally refreshed as I come out of this relaxed state....Two, I am full of energy as I open my eyes....Three, I am now closer to my goal in my conscious state. I move closer to success'.[5]

> "Begin to act as if you expected success, happiness and abundance" – Florence Scovel Shinn

In the book 'Mind Gym-An Athlete's Guide to Inner Excellence' by Gary Mack and David Casstevens, they describe the A.C.T. exercise. It says, A-Accept your present situation and understand your strengths and weaknesses. C-Create your desired state, closing your eyes, see where you want to be, then write it down. T-Take action through goal setting and success is taking one step at a time.[6]

Looking in the Mirror
Looking in the mirror is a self-awareness exercise, but it can also help you to discern and visualise what you really want for yourself. Look into your eyes and reflect on your life and think what you really want. Spend a number of minutes doing this and it will help establish your goals clearly.

The Foundations of wellbeing

To improve health and wellbeing, you need to focus on the **Four Daily Cornerstones:**

1. To eat nutritious, healthy food mindfully.
2. To exercise mindfully, engaging in a target level of physical exercise every day.
3. Practicing some mind body exercise each day, e.g. meditation, Tai chi, Qi Gong, yoga etc to reduce stress levels and cortisol.
4. To establish better sleep patterns; going to bed earlier and doing some meditation when you find it hard to sleep.

The Chinese Body-clock – The Circadian rhythms

In Traditional Chinese Medicine, there is an optimal time for every activity, during the day and night. It is like an internal self-care body clock regulating the organs of the body. However it is up to us to get in sync with this body clock, by self-discipline and focus. By developing an awareness of our body-clock, we can begin to understand any imbalances in the body.

Circadian rhythms are the changes, physical, mental and behavioural that follow a daily cycle. The main factor influencing Circadian rhythms is daylight. Circadian rhythms affect sleeping and waking cycles, our eating habits, hormone release and body temperature. If we are consistently following poor sleeping habits, we are putting our whole system out of balance. Having a good circadian rhythm reaps health benefits. Exposure to daylight outdoors is also good for the circadian rhythms.[7]

Circadian Clock

1am–3am
The Liver
– Rest and deep sleep, blood detoxification

3am–5am
The Lungs
– Detox lungs, deep sleep, memory and dreams

5am–7am
Large Intestine
– Waking up, bowel movement, meditating

7am–9am
The Stomach
– Eat breakfast, good time to concentrate, physical exercise

9am–11am
The Spleen
– Spleen converts food to Qi, clear thinking

11am–1pm
The Heart
– Eat lunch, good energy, blood circulation

1pm–3pm
The Small Intestine
– Sorting and absorbing food, lower energy, good time to nap

3pm–5pm
The Bladder
– Energy revives, waste released, good time for work and study

5pm–7pm
The Kidney
– Suppertime, body stores nutrients and builds bone marrow

7pm–9pm
The Pericardium
– Time for self-love, protection and light reading

9pm–11pm
Triple Burner
– Rest and getting to sleep, metabolic and endocrine balancing

11pm–1am
Gallbladder – Sleep, building blood Cells, cellular repair, releasing bile.[8]

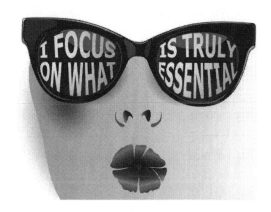

CHAPTER TWELVE

Recipes and Remedies

....

Breakfast muesli
2 cups of rolled oats
Half a cup of sunflower and pumpkin seeds
Add chopped apricots and dates
A dessertspoon of flaxseed
Half a cup of chopped strawberries and blueberries
Add almond milk or orange juice

Oatmeal with raisins
2 cups of rolled oats
Half a cup of raisins
3 cups of water
2 pinches of sea salt

Method:
Heat a wok or stainless steel pan. Add dry oats, turn to low heat, roast oats slowly and stir constantly to avoid burning. Take off heat when roasted. Put oats in pot and add raisins, water and salt. Cover and bring to boil. Simmer on low heat for 25 to 30 minutes. Then add barley malt or honey and seeds of choice.

Buck wheat pancakes

One cup of buckwheat flour
Half a cup of whole wheat flour
Pinch of salt
One cup of water or apple juice
Small amount of sesame oil

Method:
Mix the dry ingredients. Add water or apple juice. Mix with spoon. Allow batter to sit overnight in a warm place so it starts to ferment. Lightly oil a pan with sesame oil. Place batter on pan. Cook over medium heat until lightly brown. Turn pancake over and fry until golden brown.

Berry and Banana smoothie

One banana chopped
One cup berries frozen or fresh
Add water or almond milk(unsweetened)
Whisk in Blender

Carrot and apple smoothie

Grate one inch of ginger
3 to 4 large carrots chopped
2 small apples chopped
One stick of celery chopped
Add water or unsweetened almond milk
Whisk in blender

Trail mix for morning and afternoon snacks

Pumpkin and sunflower seeds
Dried fruit – cranberries and chopped dates or figs
Chopped walnuts and almonds

Mix in bowl and divide into two or three small bags to carry with you on the go.

Salads
Healthy Salad lunch
Handful of leaf spinach chopped
Handful of rocket leaves
Half onion chopped
Half red/or yellow pepper chopped
Two inches of cucumber sliced
One carrot chopped
Half cup of red cabbage chopped
Two avocados sliced
4 /5 cherry tomatoes
Drizzle with small amount of apple cider vinegar and lemon juice

Quick and easy salad
One cup spinach
Half a cup of rocket leaves
Small can of tuna or mackerel
One avocado sliced
Boiled egg sliced

Drizzle with tablespoon of apple cider vinegar and one dessertspoon of low fat mayonnaise to taste

Oriental rice salad
125g brown rice
2tbsp sesame oil
2tbsp lime juice
20g sunflower seeds

50 g sesame seeds
1 dessert spoon grated ginger
2 tablespoons of lime or lemon juice
Pinch ground black pepper

Method:
Cook brown rice in water. When tender, drain well. Add sesame oil, ginger, and lime juice while still warm. Allow to cool. Toast seeds in a grill or oven until brown. Add seeds to rice and pinch of black pepper

Soups
Kombu dashi stock
This seaweed-mushroom stock can be used for miso soup.
Ingredients:
3 to four dried shitake mushrooms
2 to 3 5-inch square pieces of kombu (Japanese seaweed)
1 tsp of salt
3 and a half pints of water

Method:
In a pot add mushrooms, kombu, water, salt. Boil, lower the heat and simmer for 30 mins.

Miso soup
Ingredients:
2 cups of seaweed-mushroom stock
one cup combination of mushrooms, tofu, finely chopped cabbage and wakame seaweed rehydrated
4 tsp miso

Method:
Bring stock to a simmer. In a separate pan heat and cook

mushrooms, tofu and vegetables in oil until ready. Add chopped vegetables, mushrooms, tofu and seaweed to stock and cook for three to four minutes. Remove from the heat. Whisk the miso and two tablespoons of stock. Add miso and stock back into soup and stir well. Serve and enjoy!

Easy Miso soup
Ingredients:
One pint of water
Add two cubes of vegetable stock
Add chopped nori seaweed sheet and add one large mug of finely chopped green cabbage, onion and tofu to the soup and bring to boil and allow to simmer for 15 minutes. Whisk 4 tsp miso in hot water to get smooth mixture. Remove soup from heat and stir in miso! serve and enjoy!

Lentil soup
Ingredients:
One cup of diced onions
One cup of sliced celery
One cup of green lentils
6 to 7 cups of water
One cup of noodles
One cup of finely chopped carrots
One quarter cup of chopped parsley as garnish

Place all ingredients in a pot except noodles and parsley. Cover and bring to boil, then let simmer for 30 minutes. Add noodles and simmer for 5 mins or until noodles are tender. Serve and garnish with the chopped parsley.

Noodles and broth
Ingredients:
One packet of buckwheat noodles
5 inch strip of Kombu
2 shiitake mushrooms
3 tablespoons of soy sauce
2 to three inches of ginger root grated
6 cups of water
One sheet of Nori

Method:
Cook Noodles in water and drain when cooked. Put 2 cups of water in a pot and bring to boil, add the chopped shiitake mushrooms, chopped nori, chopped kombu, shoyu and grated ginger to boiling water, cover pot and simmer for 15 minutes. Add noodles.

Healthy soup
Ingredients:
3 to 4 stalks of celery sliced
2 cloves of chopped garlic
2 small leeks or onions sliced
454g of chopped tomatoes
454g of potatoes sliced

Cover with water. Add one cube of vegetable stock. Sprinkle with dried or fresh parsley and oregano. Bring to boil and simmer.

Serve and enjoy. If you prefer a smooth soup you can whisk it smooth. Refrigerate leftovers for use the next day!

Main Meals
Bulghur and vegetables
Ingredients:
3 cups of bulghur
5 cups of water
1 cup of onions sliced
Half a cup of carrots diced
Half a cup of celery diced
Chopped parsley
A pinch of salt

Method:
Put water in pot, add carrots, celery and salt, bring to boil and then simmer for 15 minutes. Remove pot from cooker and add the bulghur. Close lid and leave to sit for 10 to 15 minutes until water is absorbed, mix together and serve with parsley.

Organic chicken stir-fry
Ingredients:
350gr of organic chicken breast cut into strips
2 large carrots finely chopped
1 to 2 cloves of garlic chopped
One pepper chopped
2 to 3 sticks of celery sliced
One onion sliced
75g of mangetout
One tablespoon of oil
100g of beansprouts
2 tablespoons of soy sauce

Method:
Heat oil in frying pan or wok. Add chicken and cook for 5

minutes. Add carrots, onion, celery, peppers to chicken and cook for 7 to 8 minutes. Add remaining ingredients and stir all together for another 5 to 6 minutes. Serve with brown rice

Prawn chow mein
Ingredients:
One green pepper sliced
One onion sliced
2 sticks of celery chopped
120g bean sprouts
2 tablespoons of soy sauce
200g mushrooms sliced
225g prawns
350ml of tomato juice
2 tablespoons of lemon juice

Method:
Heat tomato juice, lemon juice and soy sauce in a pan. Add all the vegetables except sprouts. Boil all together and simmer for 15 minutes. Cook prawns in wok for ten minutes with oil. Add sprouts for last 3 minutes. Add cooked prawns and sprouts to pan of tomato juice and vegetables, stir for 3 minutes and serve with brown rice or noodles.

Ginger and almond stir fry
Ingredients:
4oz flaked almonds
2 inch piece of sliced fresh ginger
2 crushed or sliced garlic cloves
Sliced spring onions
One pepper sliced into small pieces
4oz courgettes

Packet of tofu cut into cubes
4oz mangetout
4oz mushrooms
1 tsp sesame oil
2 dessertspoons of olive oil
2 dessertspoons cornflour
One and a half cups of vegetable stock
2 dessertspoons of basil
2 dessertspoons parsley
Pinch of ground black pepper
Tablespoon of soya sauce

Method:
Toast almonds. In a frying pan or wok heat the sesame and olive oil. Add ginger and garlic. Add chopped vegetables, stirring while cooking. Add tofu. In separate pot mix cornflour and vegetable stock until smooth. Add to frying pan or wok. Add herbs and toasted almonds. Bring to boil, stirring and then let simmer until vegetables tender and cooked. Serve with brown rice.

Japanese vegetable noodles with tofu
Ingredients:
120g soba noodles
1 tablespoon dark soy sauce
1 tablespoon Japanese rice wine
1 tsp of sesame oil
80g mangetout
1 courgette sliced fully

For the tofu
3cm ginger grated
1 clove garlic chopped

1 red chilli
2 tsp soya sauce
2 tablespoons of preferred oil
180g tofu cut into pieces

Method:
Steam all the vegetables. Bring water to boil in large pan. Add soba noodles and boil for 5 minutes. Drain and rinse. Put noodles back in pan with rest of noodle ingredients. In a bowl mix ginger, garlic, chilli and soy sauce. In frying pan or wok put oil of choice. Fry tofu for 3 mins after dabbing with kitchen towel before putting in pan. Spoon the garlic ginger sauce over tofu and serve with noodles.

Lentil and walnut burgers
Ingredients:
2 garlic cloves crushed or sliced
170g red split lentils
420ml water
2 small onions chopped
1 tsp thyme
1 tsp oregano
3 tablespoons tomato puree
Pinch ground black pepper
120g chopped walnuts
1 tablespoon of sunflower seeds
Small amount of rice flour for coating
Olive oil for coating

Method:
Put onions, garlic, lentils, water and herbs into saucepan and bring to boil. Simmer, stir occasionally until lentils soft for 35 minutes.

Drain water. Stir in tomato puree and chopped walnuts
Add pinch of black pepper. Allow to cool. Sprinkle rice flour
with sesame seeds on work surface. Divide mixture into six
Roll each piece into seeds and flour. Flatten each portion
into burger shape. Brush portions with olive oil and bake for
approximately 25 minutes at 200 degrees centigrade.

Sushi
Ingredients:
5 to 6 sheets of Nori
2 cups of brown rice
2 and a half cups of water
1 carrot cut in strips
2 scallions cut in pieces
One quarter jar of miso chutney

Method:
Cook rice. Slice a carrot into strips and chop in pieces and
put in boiling water for three minutes. Grill nori sheet under
strong heat until it turns dark green. Take out from grill.
Place on chopping board and spread the rice evenly on the

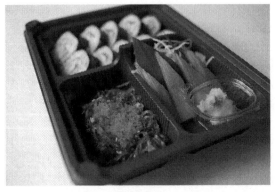

Sushi box

nori sheet. Leave one inch of nori uncovered at end furthest away from you and one quarter inch at end nearest to you· The vegetables are placed on edge/end nearest to you with half a teaspoon of miso chutney on top of them. Roll the contents in the sushi mat into a log shape, wet the edge / end furthest away to seal. Tidy up the ends and cut into one inch thick slices to serve.

Desserts

Fruit salad with apple and cinnamon sauce
Ingredients:
Chop one apple into pieces
Slice a banana and pear
Small portion of grapes

For sauce:
Mix 250ml of apple juice, 5 tablespoons of tahini and one teaspoon of cinnamon in blender until smooth. Pour mixture over fruit in a bowl. Enjoy!

Mango and orange slushy sorbet
Ingredients:
2 large mangoes
140ml orange juice

Method:
Peel and pit mangoes and dice. Place sliced mango on tray and freeze until solid. Put orange juice in fridge to cool. Put frozen mango and orange juice in blender, whisk until smooth. Serve and enjoy!

Caremelized bananas

Ingredients:

One quarter cup of brown sugar

One quarter cup of water

Two bananas halved lengthwise

Method:

In small frying pan over low to medium heat mix water and sugar. Stir until sugar is dissolved. Add bananas, cook for 6 minutes. Then turn bananas and cook other side for four to five minutes. Enjoy!

Teas and Remedies

Bancha Tea

Bancha tea is helpful in strengthening the metabolism when fatigued or ill. Use one table spoon of tea to four cups of water. Bring tea to the boil and then reduce the temperature and allow to simmer for no more than four or five minutes. Drink two to three times a day.

Dandelion Root Tea

Dandelion root tea helps to strengthen the heart and small intestine. Mix one tablespoon of dried dandelion root to four cups of water and bring to the boil. Reduce heat and simmer for ten minutes.

Green Tea

Green tea has many benefits. Not only does it assist the metabolism, it also helps discharge excess cholesterol. To make, put half a teaspoon in a teapot. Pour in one cup of boiling water and allow to steep. Strain and drink.

Kombu Tea

Kombu Tea helps to improve the quality of the blood and remineralizes the body. Place a three to four inch strip of Kombu sea vegetable in four cups of water. Bring to the boil, reduce the heat and simmer for ten minutes. Remove the Kombu and serve.

Lotus Root Tea

This Tea is helpful in relieving coughs and mucus in the lungs. Add two tablespoons of lotus root to one cup of water. Bring to the boil, reduce the heat and simmer for ten to fifteen minutes. Add a pinch of salt and drink.

Morning Detox Drink

Apple cider vinegar – 2 tablespoons
Lemon juice – 2 tablespoons
Honey – 1 tablespoon
Cinnamon – 1 teaspoon
Water – 1 glass

Ginger Compress

Good for coughs and mucus. You need a piece of cheesecloth or cotton and some sticking plaster. In a cup mix one teaspoon of honey, a dessertspoon of olive oil, one dessertspoon of arrowroot powder, one tablespoon of grated ginger root or ginger powder. Place the mixture on the cheesecloth or cotton and apply to the chest. Leave for fifteen to thirty minutes until warmed by the body.

Lotus Root Plaster

Lotus Root plaster helps move stagnated mucus from the chest. To prepare, mix one part of freshly grated ginger with sixteen parts freshly grated lotus root and three parts of flour. Spread a half inch layer on a piece of cotton gauze and place the side with the lotus root on the affected area. Leave the plaster on for several hours. The Ginger Compress above can be applied before using the lotus root plaster to help circulation and to loosen the mucus.

Thyme Foot Talc Ingredients
Mix Together:
One tablespoon of cornflour or one tablespoon of maize flour
One teaspoon of bicarbonate of soda
One teaspoon of finely powdered thyme

For Athlete's Foot:
Rub the feet and especially between the toes with lemon peel and then dust the feet with the Thyme Foot Talc above.

Mustard Seed Foot Bath
Good for tired, sweaty feet. Put two teaspoons of ground mustard powder into ten cups of warm water in a basin. Soak for 20 minutes. Relax and allow the warmth to ease your feet. Dry well and keep feet warm afterwards.

Natural Toothpaste
Ingredients:
One teaspoon of fresh sage
2 teaspoons of salt
One teaspoon of bicarbonate of soda
A quarter teaspoon of ground cloves(optional).

Grind all ingredients together until they form a fine powder. Put in a clean small jar and place lid on it. To use put a small amount on your tooth brush. Rinse your mouth with water. If you have sore gums add cloves to act as an analgesic.

References

Chapter one – Self-Care

1. Article in *Advances in Psychiatric Treatment*, volume 11, issue 5, September 2005. The emotional and physical benefits of expressive writing.
2. *Neijing – The Yellow Emperor's Classic of Medicine*.
3. Pg 115. *The Practices of Happiness, Political Economy and Wellbeing*. Edited by John Atherton, Elaine Graham and Ian Steedman. Published 2001 by Routledge.
4. *The Power of Positive Thinking*. Cedar Books/Vermillion; new edn Edition (21 May 1990).
5. www.sciencedirect.com. (Article from *Integrative Medicine Research*, Vol. 5, issue 2, June 2016, Pg 151–160).

Chapter Two – Emotions

1. *Secrets of Self-Healing* by Dr Maoshing Ni. Published by Avery (Penguin Group) 2008. Pg 29.
2. *The Foundations of Chinese Medicine* by Giovanni Maciocia. Published by Churchill Livingstone. First Published 1989. Reprinted 1995. Pg 130–132.
3. *Self Mastery Through Conscious Autosuggestion* by Emile Coue. First published 1920.
4. Article – Addicted to Fat: Overeating may alter the brain as much as Hard Drugs by Katie Harmon, *Scientific American*, March 28, 2010.
5. *The Foundations of Chinese Medicine* by Giovanni Maciocia. Published by Churchill Livingstone. First Published 1989. Reprinted 1995. Pg 129–132.
6. *Psychoneuroimmunology*. Publisher, Academic Press Inc; 2nd Revised edition (1 Jan. 1991).

7. Article – *European Journal of Integrative Medicine*. Volume 7, issue 3, May 2015, Pg 194–201. www.sciencedirect.com.
8. *Fat Around the Middle* by Marilyn Glenville. Published by Kyle Cathie Limited, 2006. Pg 12–13.
9. ABC News (Article – "Belly Fat is bad for your heart researchers say" by Dr Kelly Arps, 20 April, 2018).
10. *Fat Around the Middle* by Marilyn Glenville. Published by Kyle Cathie Limited, 2006. Pg 30–48.
11. *Frontiers in Immunology*, 16 August 2019 – How the Interplay between commensal microbiota, gut barrier integrity and mucosal immunity regulates brain immunity.
12. Article in *Scientific American* dated February 12, 2010 by Adam Hadhazy – Think twice how the guts second brain influences mood and well being.
13. Article – Your gut bacteria may make it harder to lose weight by Rachel Rettner, August 1, 2018 on www.livescience.com.
14. Article – How your gut bacteria can influence your weight – reviewed by Ruairi Robertson PhD, published on February 13, 2018 – see www.healthline.com.
15. Article – will stress injure your gut by Emily Deans, posted on 24 November 2011 on www.psychologytoday.com.
16. *Perfect Digestion* by Dr Deepak Chopra, published by Rider Press in 1995. Pg 64–65.
17. Time.com article – What's the best time to sleep by Markham Heid, updated April 27, 2017.
18. Article – Exercising to relax, Harvard Health Publishing, article updated July 13, 2018, see www.healthharvard.edu.

Chapter 3 – Diet and Nutrition

1. *Complete Chinese Medicine* by Tom Williams PhD, Published by Mustard, 1999. Pg 218–219.
2. Article dated 20 July 2011, *The Daily Mail* – Chew each mouthful 40 times to lose weight.
3. *Secrets of Self Healing* by Maoshing Ni. Published by Avery (Penguin) 2008. Page 72.
4. *Complete Chinese Medicine* by Tom Williams Ph.D. Published

by Mustard, 1999. Pg 220–221.

5. *Secrets of Self Healing* by Maoshing Ni. Published by Avery (Penguin) 2008. Pg 73–76.

6. *Fat Around the Middle* by Marilyn Glenville Ph.D. Published by Kyle Cathie Limited. Pg 60–64.

7. *Fat Around the Middle* by Marilyn Glenville Ph.D. Published by Kyle Cathie Limited. Pg 63–68.

8. *Fat Around the Middle* by Marilyn Glenville Ph.D. Published by Kyle Cathie Limited. Pg 63–68.

9. *The Macrobiotic Way* by Michio Kushi. Published by Avery (Penguin) 2004. Pg 47.

Chapter 4 – Chinese Medicine

1. *Chinese Acupuncture and Moxibustion*. Foreign Languages Press, Beijing, 1996. Pg 12–18.

2. *Chinese Acupuncture and Moxibustion*. Foreign Languages Press, Beijing, 1996. Pg 12–18.

3. *Chinese Acupuncture and Moxibustion*. Foreign Languages Press, Beijing, 1996. Pg 14.

4. *Traditional Chinese Medicine for Women* by Xiaolan Zhao. Published by Virago, 7 Sept 2006. Pg 5–7.

5. *The Foundations of Chinese Medicine* by Giovanni Maciocia. Published by Churchill Livingstone, 1995. Pg 5–7.

6. *Traditional Chinese Medicine for Women* by Xiaolan Zhao. Published by Virago, 7 Sept 2006. Pg 7.

7. *The Foundations of Chinese Medicine* by Giovanni Maciocia. Published by Churchill Livingstone, 1995. Pg 36–46.

8. *Chinese Acupuncture and Moxibustion*. Foreign Languages Press, Beijing, 1996. Pg 48.

9. *The Foundations of Chinese Medicine* by Giovanni Maciocia. Published by Churchill Livingstone, 1995. Pg 41–46.

10. *Complete Chinese Medicine* by Tom Williams Ph.D. Published by Mustard 1999. Pg 33.

11. *The Foundations of Chinese Medicine* by Giovanni Maciocia. Published by Churchill Livingstone, 1995. Pg 38–41.

12. *The Foundations of Chinese Medicine* by Giovanni Maciocia.

Published by Churchill Livingstone, 1995. Pg 72–73.

13. *Complete Chinese Medicine* by Tom Williams Ph.D. Published by Mustard 1999. Pg 44.

14. *Traditional Chinese Medicine for Women* by Xiaolan Zhao. Published by Virago, 7 Sept 2006. Pg 10.

15. *Chinese Acupuncture and Moxibustion.* Foreign Languages Press, Beijing, 1996. Pg 25.

16. *Traditional Chinese Medicine for Women* by Xiaolan Zhao. Published by Virago, 7 Sept, 2006. Pg 12–13.

17. *Complete Chinese Medicine* by Tom Williams Ph.D. Published by Mustard 1999. Pg 78.

18. Article – www.acupuncturetoday.com –"TCM and Weight Management" 24 August 2010, by Tyehao Lu, LAC, MAOM.

19. *The Foundations of Chinese Medicine* by Giovanni Maciocia. Published by Churchill Livingstone, 1995. Pg 50.

Chapter 5 – Acupuncture

1. W.H.O. From The World Health Organisation Report – Acupuncture Review and Analysis of Reports on Controlled Trials – Dr Xiaorui Zhang.

2. *The Foundations of Chinese Medicine* by Giovanni Maciocia. Published by Churchill Livingstone 1995. Pg 150.

3. *Chinese Acupuncture and Moxibustion.* Published by Foreign Languages Press, Beijing, 1996. Pg 346.

4. *Chinese Acupuncture and Moxibustion.* Published by Foreign Languages Press, Beijing, 1996. Pg 340.

5. Open Access *Maced J Med Sci.* 2015 Mar 15; 3(1): 85–90.

6. Article – "Acupuncture on Obesity Clinical Evidence and Possible Neuroendocrine Mechanisms" on 14 June 2018 in *Evidence based Complementary and Alternative Medicine* –www.ncbi.nlm.nih.gov.

7. *The Foundations of Chinese Medicine* by Giovanni Maciocia. Published by Churchill Livingstone 1995. Pg 330.

8. *The Foundations of Chinese Medicine* by Giovanni Maciocia. Published by Churchill Livingstone 1995. Pg 7.

9. *The Foundations of Chinese Medicine* by Giovanni Maciocia.

Published by Churchill Livingstone 1995. Pg 14.

10. *Chinese Acupuncture and Moxibustion*. Published by Foreign Languages Press, Beijing, 1996. Pg 244–245.

11. *The Foundations of Chinese Medicine* by Giovanni Maciocia. Published by Churchill Livingstone 1995. Pg 71–101.

Chapter six – Acupressure

Reference Books:

1. *Complete Chinese Medicine* by Tom Williams Ph.D. Published by Mustard 1999.

2. *Chinese Medicine – The Web That Has No Weaver* by Ted J. Kaptchuk.

3. *Acupressure – How to cure Ailments the Natural Way* by Michael Reed Gach. Published by Judy Piatkus Publishers Ltd. 2001.

4. *Relieving Pain with Acupressure* by Dagmar-Pauline Heinke. Published 1998 by Sterling Publishing Company Inc.

Chapter Seven – Tai chi and Qi Gong

1. *Tai Chi for Health* by Grandmaster Chen Zhenglei and Grandmaster Liming Yue. Published by Chen style Tai Chi Centre UK 2005. Pg 21–31.

2. Article – The health benefits of Tai Chi updated, August 20, 2019. Harvard Health Publishing www.healthharvard.edu.

3. Article – Journal of Clinical Psychology, volume 74, issue 1. First published, 13 June 2017. doi.org/10.1002/jclp.22482.

4. *Teaching Tai Chi effectively* by Dr Paul Lam. Published by Tai Chi Productions 2011. Pg 106–107.

5. Article – Department of Sport Science and Physical Education, the Chinese University of Hong Kong. 13 May 2015. www. hindawi.com, volume 2015, article ID976123.

6. *Tai Chi for Health* by Grandmaster Chen Zhenglei and Grandmaster Liming Yue. Published by Chen style Tai Chi Centre UK. 2005. Pg 21–33.

7. Article – *Neurorehabilitation and Neural Repair* 2018, vol. 32(2) 142–149.

8. Article – *BMJ*, 2018;360;K851.
9. Article – *Focus* 2018; 16: 40–47, doi10.1176/appi.focus. 20170042.
10. *Teaching Tai Chi effectively* by Dr Paul Lam. Published by Tai Chi Productions 2011. Pg 100.
11. Liu, Tian jun; Qiang, xiao Mei, (Eds 2013) *Chinese medical Qi Gong*, third edition. Singing Dragon. ISBN 978-1848190962.
12. *Complete Chinese Medicine* by Tom Williams Ph.D. Published by Mustard 1999. Pg 190–191.
13. *Ba Duan Jin*, Compiled by the Chinese Health Qigong Association. Published by Foreign Languages Press, Beijing, China. Third Print 2009.
14. *Ba Duan Jin*, Compiled by the Chinese Health Qi Gong Association. Published by Foreign Languages Press, Beijing, China. Third Print 2009. Pg 21–54.

Chapter Eight – Meditation

1. *The Relaxation Response* by Dr Herbert Benson. Published by Avon Books; Revised edition (1 Feb. 2000).
2. *Teach Yourself Meditation* by James Hewitt. Published by Hodder and Stoughton Educational. Eight Impression 1989. Pg 18-76.
3. *The Secrets of Chinese Meditation* by Lu K'uan Yu. Published by Samuel Weiser, Inc.
4. *Zen Training* by Katsuki Sekida. Published by Shambhala; First Edition, Sept 13, 2005.
5. *Mindfulness – A Practical Guide to Finding Peace in a Frantic World* by Mark Williams and Danny Penman. Published by Piatkus 2011. Pg 37.
6. *Understanding Meditation* by Naomi Humphrey. Published by Thorsons 1998. Pg 40–41.
7. *Peace is Every Step* by Thich Nhat Hanh. Published by Bantam Books, 1992. Pg 23.
8. *Journey into Mindfulness* by Dr Patrizia Collard. Pg 137–138.
9. Mindfulness – A practical guide to Finding Peace in a Frantic World by Mark Williams and Danny Penman. Published by Piaktus 2011. Pg 51.

10. *Mindfulness – A Practical Guide to Finding Peace in a Frantic World* by Mark Williams and Danny Penman. Published by Piaktus 2011. Pg 211–212.

Chapter Nine – The Lungs

1. *The Foundations of Chinese Medicine* by Giovanni Maciocia. Published by Churchill Livingstone. Reprinted 1995. Pg 83–87.
2. *The Foundations of Chinese Medicine* by Giovanni Maciocia. Published by Churchill Livingstone. Reprinted 1995. Pg 231–232.
3. Article – www.TheChalkboardmag.com – 13 ways to improve your Lung health according to Chinese Medicine by Mona Dan, 19/8/2019.

Chapter Ten – Herbs and Supplements

1. Article – www.healthline.com –13 potential health benefits of Dandelion. 18 July, 2018.
2. Article – www.healthline.com – 7 science based benefits of milk thistle. January 19, 2018.
3. Article – www.healthline.com –7 surprising health benefits of eating seaweed. 28 May, 2018.
4. Article – www.healthline.com – 10 proven health benefits of Turmeric and Curcumin. 13 July, 2018.
5. *Secrets of Self-Healing* by Maoshing Ni. Published by Avery (Penguin) 2008. Pg 91–97.
6. Article – www.healthline.com – 9 benefits of Co enzyme- 10. October 12, 2017.
7. *Secrets of Self-Healing* by Maoshing Ni. Published by Avery (Penguin) 2008. Pg 100–102.

Chapter Eleven –Visualisation and Goals

1. Four Tips To Visualise – www.jackcanfield.com
2. *Success Through A Positive Mental Attitude* by Napolean Hill and W. Clement Stone. Published by Thorsons 1990. Pg 67–82.
3. *Infinite Possibilities – The Art of Living Your Dreams* by Mike

Dooley, Beyond Words, Atria Paperback published 2010. Pg 23–25.

4. *Self Mastery Through Conscious Autosuggestion* by Emile Coue. Published 1920.
5. www.self-help-and-self-development.com – How to use Hypnosis for Self-Development.
6. *Mind Gym – An Athlete's Guide to Inner Excellence* by Gary Mack and David Casstevens. Published by Contemporary Books 2001.
7. Article – www.nigms.nih.gov, What are Circadian Rhythms?
8. Article – www.chalkboardmag.com. Meet the Chinese Bodyclock; is this the reason you're waking up at night? Published 30.10.17

Chapter Twelve – Recipes and Remedies

Recommended Reading:

1. *The Complete Macrobiotic Diet* by Denny Waxman. Published by Pegasus Books, 2015.
2. *The Ultimate Guide to Eating for Longevity* by Danny Waxman, Susan Waxman and Colin T. Campbell. Published by Pegasus Books, 2019.
3. *The Hip Chick's Guide to Macrobiotics* by Jessica Porter. Published by Avery 2004.
4. *Complete Guide to Macrobiotic Cooking* by Aveline Kushi, Alex Jack. Published by Grand Central Publishing, 1988.
5. *Natural Healing Through Macrobiotics* by Michio Kushi. Published by Japan Publications, 1979.
6. *Complete Chinese Cookbook* by Ken Hom. Published by BBC books 2011.
7. *The China Study Cookbook* by LeAnne Campbell, Ph.D. Published by BanBella Books, Revised Edition, 2018.
8. *Japanese Cooking, A Simple Art* by Shizuo Tsuji. Published by Kodansha Amer Inc, Reprinted 2012.
9. *The Just Bento Cookbook, Everyday Lunches to Go* by Makiko Itoh. Published by Kodansha USA. Reprinted, 2011.

Useful Contacts

U.K. AND IRELAND

Acupuncture U.K.

www.acupuncturesociety.org.uk
The Acupuncture Society
Phone: 0773 4668402
Email: acusoc@yahoo.co.uk

www.britishacupuncturefederation.co.uk
British Acupuncture Federation
197, 60 Water Ln
Wilmslow
SK9 5AJ
Phone: 0843 507 0123

The British Acupuncture Council,
www.acupuncture.org.uk
63, Jeddo Road
London
W12 9HQ
Email: info@acupuncture.org.uk
Phone: 020 8735 0400

www.medical-acupuncture.co.uk
British Medical Acupuncture Society
BMAS London
Royal London Hospital for Integrated Medicine
60 Great Ormond Street,
London WC1N 3HR
Phone: 020 7713 9437

www.aacp.org.uk
Acupuncture Association of Chartered Physiotherapists (AACP)
Sefton House, Adam Court
Newark Rd
Peterborough
PE1 5PP
U.K.
Phone: 01733 390007

www.bawma.co.uk
British Academy of Western Medical Acupuncture (BAWMA)
Phone: 07792 553429

www.bodyharmonics.co.uk
54 Fleckers
Cheltenham
GL51 3BD
U.K.
Phone: 01242 582168

Association of Traditional Chinese Medicine and Acupuncture
www.atcm.co.uk
ATCM Suite 1
The Brentano Suite
Solar House, 915 High Road
London
N12 8QJ
U.K.
Phone: 0208 457 2560

www.britishacupunctureassociation.co.uk
British Acupuncture Association
Suite 197, 60 Water Lane
Wilmslow
Cheshire
SK9 5AJ
U.K.
Phone: 0843 507 0123

Register of Chinese Herbal Medicine
The Register of Chinese Herbal Medicine, Room 1
40 Elm Hill
Norwich
NR3 1HG
Phone: 03 333 707945
www.rchm.co.uk

Acupuncture Associations Ireland

Acupuncture Council of Ireland (ACI)
www.acupuncturecouncilofireland.com
The Willows
Killballyowen
Bruff
Co. Limerick
Phone 085 8593818
Email: info@tcmci.ie

Acupuncture Foundation Professional Association(AFPA)
117 Esmondale, Naas
Co. Kildare
W91 P658
Phone: 01-4124917
Email:info@afpa.ie
www.afpa.ie

Professional Register of Traditional Chinese Medicine
PRTCM Secretary, ICTCM House, Merchants Road
Dublin 3
Phone: 01 8559000
Email: mail@prtcm.org
www.prtcm.org

European Association

European Traditional Chinese Medicine Association
www.etcma.org

U.K. Tai Chi

www.taichicentre.com
Chen Tai chi classes online and live

www.taichiunion.com
The Tai Chi union for Great Britain represents every style of Tai Chi.

www.bccma.com
They represent all the major disciplines of Chinese Martial Arts.

www.taichiforhealthinstitute.org
The Tai Chi for health Institute was founded by Dr Paul Lam and has classes and workshops worldwide.

www.yangstyletaichi.co.uk
Teaches Yang Tai Chi

www.uktaichi.com
They run classes and training courses

Tai Chi Ireland

www.westway.ie
Kevin Copeland runs Tai Chi and Qi Gong classes and also online classes

www.frankmurphysmasterclass.com
Frank Murphy Tai Chi For Health Instructor and 7th Dan Black belt IFT Tackwondo has live online classes on zoom

www.irelandtaichi.org
They have Tai Chi and Qi Gong classes and their Ireland Health Qi Gong Association runs Qi Gong Instructors Teacher Training.

www.chenireland.com
Chen Tai Chi classes

www.taichi-ireland.com
Online and live classes

www.yangfamilytaichi.ie
School for Yang Family Tai Chi Ireland

www.irishtaichi.equigeek.com
The Irish Tai Chi Chuan Association

Shiatsu U.K.
www.shiatsusociety.org
20–22 Wenlock Road
London
N1 7GU
Phone: 01788 547900

Shiatsu Ireland
www.shiatsusocietyireland.org

Macrobiotics

www.macrobiotics.org.uk
They run training classes on Macrobiotics

www.kushischool.uk
They give training classes on Macrobiotics

www.macroschool.co.uk
Run Training courses and classes

www.michelleblessing.net
Macrobiotic coaching

www.macrovegan.org

ACUPUNCTURE ORGANISATIONS U.S.A.

Accreditation Commission for Acupuncture and Oriental Medicine
www.acaom.org

American Academy of Medical Acupuncture
www.medicalacupuncture.org

American Association of Acupuncture and Oriental Medicine
www.aaaomonline.org

Council of Colleges of Acupuncture and Oriental Medicine
www.ccaom.org

National Acupuncture Detoxification Association
www.acudetox.com

National Acupuncture Foundation
www.nationalacupuncturefoundation.org

National Certification Commission for Acupuncture and Oriental Medicine
www.nccaom.org

National Federation of Chinese TCM Organisations
www.nfctcmo.org

Society for Acupuncture Research
www.acupunctureresearch.org

Traditional Chinese Medicine World Foundation
www.tcmworld.org
Acupuncture Association Europe

Tai Chi Associations U.S.A.
www.americantaichi.org
www.yangfamilytaichi.com
www.taichifoundation.org
www.ustcc.org
www.taichila.com
www.chentaichi.com
www.usataichiacademy.org
www.bodybalanceacademy.com
www.worldtaiji.com

Macrobiotics U.S.A.
www.oshawamacrobiotics.com
www.macroamerica.com
www.eastwestmacrobiotics.com
www.healingcuisine.com
www.hipchicksmacrobiotics.com
www.northbaymacro.org
www.macrobiotic.com
www.macrobioticsnewengland.com
www.clevelandmacrobiotics.org
www.strengtheninghealthinstitute.org
www.christinacooks.com
www.theblissfulchef.com
www.greatlifeglobal.com
www.thericehouse.com

Shiatsu U.S.A.
www.aobta.org

APPENDIX A

Images of Meridian Head Channels

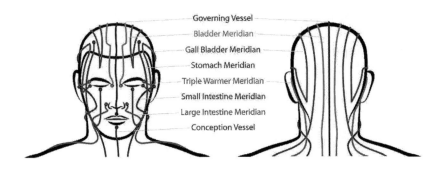

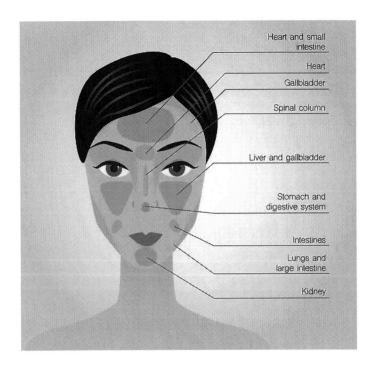

Acupuncture Ear Points

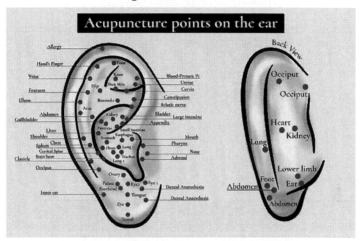

Body Meridian Channels

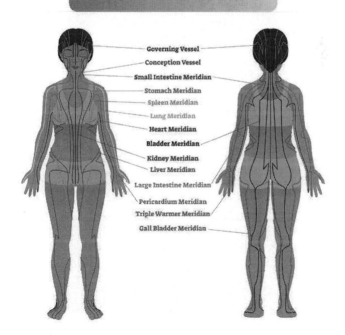

Acupuncture Model to the Rear of the Body

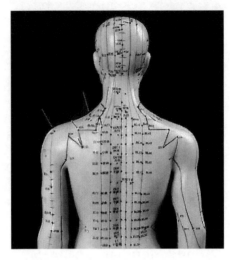

Acupuncture Model Frontal View

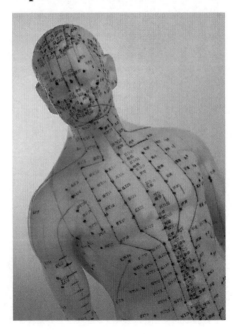

Appendix B

MACROBIOTICS

What are Macrobiotics?

Macrobiotics is a lifestyle based on harmony and balance. Macrobiotic eating places focus on healthy organic food. It also recommends no chemicals. The macrobiotic diet is predominantly vegetarian.

Macrobiotic food consists of whole grains, vegetables and other ingredients like pickles, beans, sea vegetables etc. Food preparation methods include steaming and sauteing.

The macrobiotic philosophy and diet was introduced in Japan by George Oshawa, a Japanese philosopher in the 1930's. The philosophy of macrobiotics grew in the U.S. and worldwide after the 1960's.

A macrobiotic diet is not just about food but about achieving balance in your life. Macrobiotic followers are encouraged to eat slowly, stay active and to be aware and listen to their bodies. About 50%to 60% of the daily food intake should be organically grown grains like brown rice, millet, oats and barley. Vegetables are 20%–30%of daily intake. Then 5% to 10% is bean and bean products and sea vegetables like nori agar and seaweed. Chewing food up to 30 times is recommended for good digestion. The practice of gratitude, to mindfully appreciate the gift of having food is also recommended as in Japan. Macrobiotic food is nutrient rich and low in calories. As the diet limits the consumption of fatty and sugary foods, it is complementary to a diabetic diet.

"Losing weight and then maintaining the desired weight are not difficult on the macrobiotic diet"– Michio Kushi (Founder of the Kushi Institute).

Dairy products are not generally recommended on the macrobiotic diet. The principle of Yin and Yang is part of the macrobiotic philosophy. Regular exercise is also strongly recommended in the macrobiotic lifestyle. The aim is better flexibility, increased endurance and weight management. In his book 'The Macrobiotic Way' by Michio Kushi, Michio Kushi says walking for half an hour a day will control your weight, by increasing your metabolic rate and it also helps digestion and elimination. He says it also relieves tension and worry. I have included some good macrobiotic book references in the book references section for Recipes in this book. If you are seeking further information, there are useful websites for macrobiotics in the **useful contacts section**.

"The whole point of macrobiotics is to get control of your life, and then deal with it yourself".
William Duffy (Author of – *Sugar Blues*)

**

Appendix C

SHIATSU

Shiatsu is a type of Japanese bodywork that has its origins in Traditional Chinese Medicine. In Japanese, Shiatsu means finger pressure and includes massages and assisted stretching and mobilization. A practitioner can also use palpation and pulse diagnosis. The Japanese ministry for health explains Shiatsu "as a form of manipulation by thumbs, fingers and palms without the use of instruments…to apply pressure to the human skin to correct internal malfunctions, promote and maintain health and treat specific diseases. The techniques used in Shiatsu include stretching and most commonly, leaning body weight into various points along key channels".

Shiatsu includes pressure from the thumbs and hands to the body's acupressure points and energy channels. Shiatsu is Japan's main manual therapy. There are different styles of Shiatsu, all of which originated in Japan in the early 1900's, along with a resurgence of Acupuncture. One of the principal concepts of Japanese and Chinese medicine including the practice of Shiatsu is Qi – our vital energy. You can find website details of Shiatsu associations in the U.K. Ireland and the USA in the useful contacts section of this book.

**

Appendix D

KAIZEN

Kaizen is a Japanese term that means continuous improvement. Japanese Corporations have long used the technique to achieve business goals. The Kaizen principle is to take small, but continuous steps to improvement. Robert Maurer in his book- One Small Step Can Change Your Life-The Kaizen Way, says posing Kaizen questions helps us to reach our goals e.g.:

1. If health were my first priority, what would I be doing differently today?
2. How could I incorporate a few more minutes of exercise into my daily routine?

He says that people who ordinarily would say that they have no time for their health, will start to come up with new and creative ways to establish good habits. He says that by asking small questions we will keep our fight or flight response in the off position. He gives further examples of Kaizen questions.

3. What is one small step I could take toward reaching my goal?
4. What is one small step I could do to improve my health?

Robert Maurer says by continuing to ask the same small questions, you will be programming your brain for the right solution.

> "Confront the difficult while it is still easy;accomplish the great task by a series of small acts".
> – Tao Te Ching

Robert Maurer's book *'One Small Step Can Change Your Life'* – *The Kaizen Way,* is published by Workman Publishing New York. His website is www.scienceofexcellence.com

**

Appendix E

WELLBEING ASSESSMENT

How good is your nutrition and Diet?
Poor
Average
Good
Excellent

How good is your exercise and fitness?
Poor
Average
Good
Excellent

How is your sleep?
Poor
Average
Good
Excellent

How is your emotional health and strategy for stress?
Poor
Average
Good
Excellent

How are your social and family relations?
Poor
Average
Good
Excellent

How good are you at budgeting and finances?
Poor
Average
Good
Excellent

Are you spending your time and work time in a way that aligns with your goals and values?
Poor
Average
Good
Excellent

Is your living space clutter free and safe?
Poor
Average
Good
Excellent

**

Appendix F

DAILY GOALS:

IN YOUR JOURNAL OR DIARY, LIST YOUR DAILY GOALS. USING COLOURED PENS AND PICTURES TO ENGAGE YOUR MEMORY AND MOTIVATION.

MY WEEKLY GOALS:

USING YOUR JOURNAL OR DIARY, USE COLOURED MARKERS AND PICTURES TO ENGAGE YOUR MEMORY AND MOTIVATION.

MY MONTHLY GOALS:

USING A JOURNAL OR DIARY, USE COLOURED PENS AND PICTURES TO ENGAGE YOUR MOTIVATION AND MEMORY.

Index

The Author-Caroline Rainsford
www.carolinerainsfordco.com

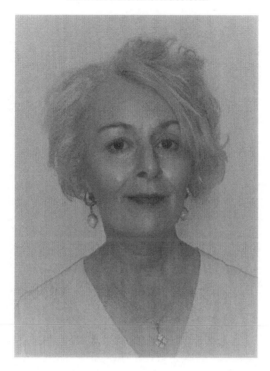

About the author: Caroline Rainsford is an Acupuncturist and trained as a Tai Chi Instructor with Dr Paul Lam of the Tai Chi for Health Institute. She has also attended workshops with Grandmasters Liming Yue and Chen Zhenglei. She has qualifications in Neuro Linguistic Programming and Hypnotherapy.She is passionate about publicising the benefits of Meditation, Qi Gong, Tai Chi, Acupuncture and Nutrition. She has an instagram page chihealthcarolinerainsford and her website is www.carolinerainsfordco.com

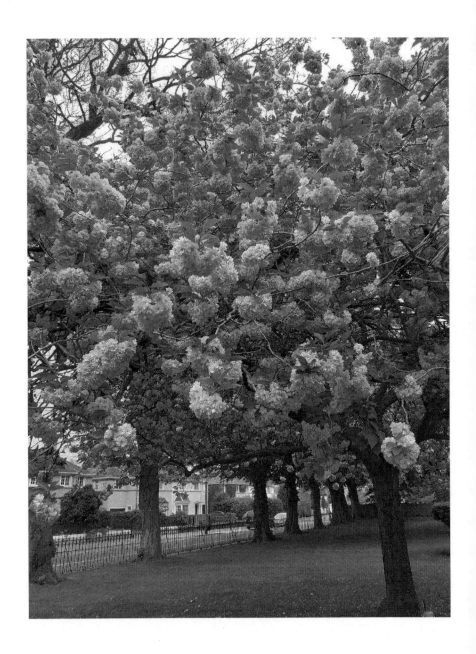